Anterolateral Rotatory Instability in ACL Deficient Knee

Andrea Ferretti
Editor

Anterolateral Rotatory Instability in ACL Deficient Knee

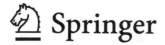 Springer

Editor
Andrea Ferretti
Department of Surgery and Translational Medicine
Sant'Andrea University Hospital, La Sapienza University
Rome, Italy

ISBN 978-3-031-00117-8   ISBN 978-3-031-00115-4   (eBook)
https://doi.org/10.1007/978-3-031-00115-4

This Springer imprint is published by the registered company Springer Nature Switzerland AG
The registered company address is: Gewerbestrasse 11, 6330 Cham, Switzerland

For my thoughts are not your thoughts or your ways my ways—Isaiah, 55; 8

To Stefania and Federico

Foreword

You will never fully understand rotatory instability as long as you look only at ACL (Andrea Ferretti)

I met Andrea Ferretti, a young resident, in the 1970s at the Orthopaedic Institute at the University of Rome where I was an Associate Professor. We worked together for almost 10 years, and like me, he was dedicated mostly to the treatment of athletes, and especially to knee surgery. His dedication to this specialty was demonstrated when, 20 years later, he was named Professor of Orthopaedics at the Sant'Andrea Hospital in Rome and Chief Doctor of the Italian Football Association and a UEFA Medical Committee member.

When Andrea invited me to write the foreword for this book, I was not only honoured, but for me, it was like a return to the past.

Since a normal sports life is impossible without proper joint function and since proper joint function cannot occur with laxity, orthopaedic surgeons need to know not only the treatments for instability but also the history of the treatments. Many facets of surgery have changed, and many others are the same. Often, the techniques of the past are abandoned, and years later, they start to be used again.

Considering the past 10 years, advances in the number and development of newer arthroscopic procedures, knee ligament reconstructions, meniscus repairs, and the treatment of articular cartilage pathology have resulted in corresponding needs for education, training, and knowledge.

All of this new knowledge introduces challenging problems for practising surgeons and to orthopaedic residents in training.

Most importantly, this knowledge provides the basis upon which an orthopaedist counsels a patient regarding the risks and benefits of every operative treatment. Many patients, before or after the physician visit, search the internet to try to understand if the suggestions of the treating surgeon are the same as those suggested by the "opinion leaders".

They often become confused and frightened by very different suggestions and proposals. These patients have high expectations for overcoming their complaints and their ability to return to their previous activity level.

The text of this book is comprehensive and covers all aspects of the anatomy and biomechanics of anterior cruciate reconstruction.

Wishing great success to Andrea Ferretti and all other authors, I would like to share four quotations, with the first from William Harvey (1578–1657): "I would say with Fabricius[1]: let all reasoning be silent when experience gainsays its conclusion. The too familiar vice of the present age is to obtrude as manifest truths, mere fancies, born of conjecture and superficial reasoning, altogether unsupported by the testimony of sense". The second is from Robert Leach: "Enjoy the book, absorb the material that was so assiduously collected by the editors and use that material to the benefit of your patients". The third quotation is from my mentor Jack C. Hughston: "To readers I would say, let the experience presented in this book speak for itself". The fourth is from Andrea Ferretti himself: "You will never fully understand rotatory instability as long as you look only at ACL".

Giancarlo Puddu

---

[1] Girolamo Fabrici d'Acquapendente (1533–1639), Surgeon, Professor of Anatomy at the University of Padua and master of dr. William Hartley

Contents

Contributors

Alessandro Annibaldi Orthopaedic Unit, Sant'Andrea University Hospital, La Sapienza University, Rome, Italy

Angelo De Carli Orthopaedic Unit, Sant'Andrea University Hospital, La Sapienza University, Rome, Rome, Italy

Alessandro Carrozzo Orthopaedic Unit, Sant'Andrea University Hospital, La Sapienza University, Rome, Italy

Fabio Conteduca Orthopaedic Unit, Sant'Andrea University Hospital, La Sapienza University, Rome, Italy

Andrea Ferretti Orthopaedic Unit, Sant'Andrea University Hospital, La Sapienza University, Rome, Italy

Orthopaedic Unit, Sant'Andrea University Hospital, La Sapienza University, Rome, Rome, Italy

Edoardo Gaj Orthopaedic Unit, Sant'Andrea University Hospital, La Sapienza University, Rome, Italy

Matteo Guzzini Orthopaedic Unit, Sant'Andrea University Hospital, La Sapienza University, Rome, Italy

Ferdinando Iannotti Orthopaedic Unit, Sant'Andrea University Hospital, La Sapienza University, Rome, Italy

Raffaele Iorio Orthopaedic Unit, Sant'Andrea University Hospital, La Sapienza University, Rome, Italy

Luca Labianca Sant'Andrea Sapienza University Hospital, Rome, Italy

Barbara Maestri Orthopaedic Unit, Sant'Andrea University Hospital, La Sapienza University, Rome, Italy

Orthopaedic Surgeon, Sant'Andrea Sapienza University Hospital, Rome, Italy

Daniele Mazza Orthopaedic Unit, Sant'Andrea University Hospital, La Sapienza University, Rome, Italy

Edoardo Monaco Orthopaedic Unit, Sant'Andrea University Hospital, La Sapienza University, Rome, Italy

Federico Morelli Orthopaedic Unit, Sant'Andrea University Hospital, La Sapienza University, Rome, Italy

Susanna M. Pagnotta Orthopaedic Unit, Sant'Andrea University Hospital, La Sapienza University, Rome, Italy

Paola Papandrea Sant'Andrea Sapienza University Hospital, Rome, Italy

Andrea Redler Orthopaedic Unit, Sant'Andrea University Hospital, La Sapienza University, Rome, Italy

Edoardo Viglietta Orthopaedic Unit, Sant'Andrea University Hospital, La Sapienza University, Rome, Italy

History of Modern ACL Surgery

1

Andrea Ferretti, Edoardo Viglietta, and Fabio Conteduca

The interest of surgeons in anterior cruciate ligament (ACL) injuries dates back to the nineteenth century, and the first surgical technique descriptions were reported at the beginning of the twentieth century. Among the pioneers of knee ligament surgery, an Italian surgeon, Riccardo Galeazzi, should be credited for the first known report of an ACL reconstruction technique using the semitendinosus tendon [1, 2] (Fig. 1.1).

However, modern ACL surgery dates back to the sixties, when rotatory instability was clearly described as the consequence of an ACL tear. In fact, some previous studies have already reported a pathological rotational phenomenon in ACL-deficient knees [3]. The comprehensive description of the pivot shift phenomenon provided in 1968 by Slocum and Larson [4] gave the crucial impulse for the development of modern ACL surgery. The new and quite surprising finding of their study consisted of the role of the ACL in controlling tibial internal rotation along with its well-known effect on tibial anterior translation. The name "pivot shift phenomenon" was ascribed to a pathological movement resulting from the increase in anterior tibial translation and tibial internal rotation of the lateral tibial plateau. This phenomenon could be clinically elicited by examining the knee with a simple manoeuvre that quickly became known as the pivot shift test. Until then, the most popular method to diagnose an ACL tear was the anterior drawer test, usually performed with 90° of knee flexion. However, the pivot shift test, whose aim was to evaluate the amount of rotatory instability, soon became a specific diagnostic test to diagnose ACL insufficiency, even when the classic anterior drawer test with 90° of knee flexion was negative.

A. Ferretti (✉) · E. Viglietta · F. Conteduca
Orthopaedic Unit, Sant'Andrea University Hospital, La Sapienza University, Rome, Italy

© The Author(s), under exclusive license to Springer Nature Switzerland AG 2022
A. Ferretti (ed.), *Anterolateral Rotatory Instability in ACL Deficient Knee*, https://doi.org/10.1007/978-3-031-00115-4_1

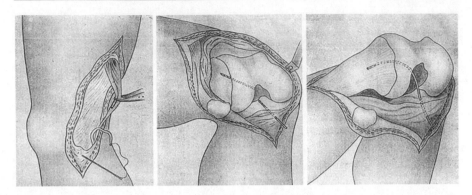

Fig. 1.1 First report on an ACL reconstruction technique using the semitendinosus tendon. Reprinted with permission from "Galeazzi R. Atti e Memorie della Società Lombarda di Chirurgia, II [1934], pp. 302–316 [2]"

Surprisingly, enough, the pivot shift test was introduced well before than the anterior drawer test with mild flexion (i.e. the Lachman test) became popular. The Lachman test was first described by Torg and coauthors [5] in 1976 and rapidly became the most specific and sensible test for the diagnosis of ACL tears, regardless of the amount of rotatory instability. However, the pivot shift test remains the best way to evaluate functional impairment in cases of ACL insufficiency, as it better correlates with the subjective feeling of instability and giving-way episodes described by patients [6].

Since its first description, many changes in how to clinically elicit the pivot shift phenomenon have been proposed by various authors. Among many propositions, it is noteworthy to mention how the "jerk test" was first described by Hughston et al. [7] in their 1976 paper:

> With the patient supine, the examiner supports the lower extremity, flexing the hip to approximately 45 degrees and the knee to 90 degrees and internally rotating the tibia. If the right knee is being examined, the examiner grasps the foot with the right hand and internally rotates the tibia while placing the left hand on the proximal end of the fibula to exert valgus stress. Then, the examiner extended the knee gradually, maintaining internal rotation and valgus stress. If the test is positive, subluxation of the lateral femorotibial joint reaches a maximum flexion at approximately 30 degrees, and then, as the right knee extends further, spontaneous relocation occurs. Relocation implies a sudden change in the relative velocities of the tibia and femur, i.e. there is a sudden change in the rate of acceleration of the two surfaces which, in engineering terminology, is called a jerk.

It is currently common practice to grade the amount of rotatory instability and the severity of the pivot shift test as mild (+−−, gliding), moderate (++−, clunk), and severe (+++, subluxation). Today, the term "explosive" pivot shift is also used to identify the most severe instabilities.

Since the mid-seventies, the concepts of rotational instability in ACL-deficient knees and the pivot shift phenomenon have run together in relation to the pathogenesis, mechanism of injury, diagnosis, treatment, and prognosis. It is now well accepted that "the goal of an ACL reconstruction should be to eliminate the pivot shift" [3].

In Italy, the jerk test was introduced and spread by Arnaldo Moschi and Giancarlo Puddu, who became familiar with it during their 1976 fellowship at the Hughston Sports Medicine Clinic in Columbus (GE). However, to the best of our knowledge, the first Italian publication in which the jerk test was described dates back to 1980 [8]. Giancarlo Puddu and Arnaldo Moschi also imported (to Italy) the classification system of ligamentous sprains and knee instability proposed by Hughston in his publication in the American Volume of Journal of Bone and Joint Surgery in March 1976 [7], where he reported the Standard Nomenclature of Athletic Injuries, as issued by the Committee on the Medical Aspects of Sports of the American Medical Association. This classification still represents a milestone for understanding the basis for the proper diagnosis and treatment of knee ligament injuries.

Ligament tears can be classified into three levels: level I consists of a "simple" stretching of the ligament that goes beyond the limit of its elasticity; level II implies a partial tear of the ligament, which is weakened but still maintains its continuity and function; and level III consists of a complete rupture of the ligament, which loses its continuity and function. While in levels I and II, the joint remains stable, level III results in instability, characterized by abnormal and excessive joint motion.

Instabilities resulting from level III ligament tears can be further divided into three grades according to the amount of joint opening: in grade I, the joint opens less than 5 millimetres; in grade II, it opens from 5 to 10 millimetres; and in grade III, it opens more than 10 millimetres. This classification is worth remembering because there is still some confusion on this subject in scientific publications, where levels of ligament tears are often mistaken with degrees of instability and partial tears are thought to result in mild instability.

The pattern of knee instability is even more interesting. The same paper by Hughston and coauthors recognized two main types of knee instability: straight (nonrotatory) or rotatory (either simple or combined). This classification is mainly based on the involvement of the posterior cruciate ligament (PCL), whose complete injury may result in straight instability (Table 1.1).

The type of instability could be identified after a series of instability tests, such as the varus and valgus stress tests, performed at either 30° of flexion or in full extension, the posterior and anterior drawer tests (the latter later replaced by the Lachman test) with the foot in neutral, internal, or external rotation, and finally the jerk test. Other less important tests were also suggested.

As a result, since the seventies, anterolateral rotatory instability (ALRI) has been associated with ACL-deficient knees and the pivot shift phenomenon.

Surprisingly, all these, old, proposed clinical classifications resulted from studies conducted over relatively small series of cases collected over several years. Indeed, in those years, knee ligament surgery was a very sophisticated and quite adventurous reconstruction procedure that was still limited to a few hyperspecialized centres around the world. Only a few knee surgery pioneers would perform quite "experimental" techniques usually for severely injured professional athletes who were willing to try anything to return to the sport. Today, we feel great admiration for these brave physicians, who, with limited resources, had extraordinary and brilliant intuitions, most of them confirmed by later studies to be based on more sophisticated technologies.

Table 1.1 Rotatory instabilities of the knee

Rotatory instability	Involved ligaments	Clinical findings
Isolated:		
– Anteromedial	MCL	Valgus stress test 30° (+)
		Anterior drawer test in ER (+)
	MCL + POL	Valgus stress test 30° (++)
		Anterior drawer test in ER (++)
– Anterolateral	ACL	Lachman test (+)
		Pivot shift test (+)
	ACL + ALL	Lachman test (+)
		Pivot shift test (++/+++)
– Posterolateral	LCL	Varus stress test 30° (+)
	LCL + arcuate complex	Varus stress test 30° (++)
		Reverse pivot shift test (+)
		Recurvatum test (+)
		Dial test 30° (+)
Combined:		
– Anteromedial & Anterolateral		
– Anteromedial & Posterolateral	}	Resulting from the combination of the findings of isolated rotatory instabilities
– Anterolateral & Posterolateral		
– Anteromedial & Anterolateral & posterolateral		

ALL Anterolateral Ligament, *LCL* Lateral Collateral Ligament, *MCL* Medial Collateral Ligament, *POL* Posterior Oblique Ligament

In fact, in addition to laboratory experiments, for a better understanding of the true pathogenesis and biomechanics of knee instabilities, only studies on surgeries carried out soon after an ACL tear had occurred (the so-called "*acute phase*") could be considered actually proving. In late surgeries, the original lesions could be masked by scar tissue, and additional lesions could originate from further joint damage occurring as an effect of new traumatic episodes or of the natural course of the instability.

In some of the first papers reporting the surgical anatomy of acute ALRI, published by Hughston and his fellows [9–11], a wide range of injuries was reported, even some cases where the ACL was not involved and apparently normal. However, thanks to the contribution of arthroscopy and related techniques, several studies have later strengthened the fact that ALRI consists of anterior subluxation of the lateral tibial plateau, which rotates internally over the lateral femoral condyle and pivots on a normal PCL. This condition, easily revealed by a positive pivot shift test, could only occur as a consequence of an ACL tear. However, since the seventies and eighties, some knee scholars, both in Europe and the USA, recognized that even though the pivot shift is due to an ACL tear and related insufficiency, it is significantly increased as a result of an associated tear of the so-called secondary restraints in the lateral compartment [7, 12, 13]. The anatomy of these structures was investigated in different ways and with conflicting results by several authors, as reported in a dedicated chapter (see Chap. 2).

The main heritage of Hughston and his fellows consists of the recognition of the role of capsular secondary restraint injuries in the pathogenesis of ALRI, which could even overcome the role of the ACL itself. Moreover, they initially supported the concept that the accurate repair/reconstruction of medial and lateral extra-articular anatomical structures was able to re-establish normal knee stability, even with a torn and unreconstructed ACL. Therefore, they set up a series of surgical techniques aimed at repairing or reinforcing the secondary restraints rather than reconstructing the ACL itself. They became popular for comparing the control of the human knee to a horse, whose movement is guided by bridles, mainly represented, in the knee, by the semimembranosus on the medial side and the biceps on the lateral side.

For several years, Hughston's principles have been carefully followed by all of us, and in ALRI, isolated extra-articular procedures such as the advancement of semimembranosus and the posterior oblique ligament (POL), medially, and the advancement of the biceps or fascia lata tenodesis, laterally, were performed (Figs. 1.2, 1.3 and 1.4).

However, the overall results of these techniques were not considered fully satisfactory. Indeed, in 1982, we published on the "Revue de Chirurgie Orthopédique" the results of extra-articular reconstructions in 48 high-level athletes [14]. After a mean follow-up of 28 months (ranging from 15 to 60 months), only 12 of the 43 patients included in the study were able to return to a preinjury level of performance, and the operation clearly failed in 13 patients. Based on these results, treatment with isolated extra-articular procedures was given up.

In November 1979, the first intra-articular reconstruction was performed at our institute by Giancarlo Puddu, using the semitendinosus as an autologous graft. The original technique, later published in the American Journal of Sports Medicine [8] and on the VIII edition of "the Bible of the Orthopaedics", the Campbell's Operative Orthopaedics, consisted of the distal detachment of the tendon from the pes anserinus, along with a small plug of bone; the tendon was carefully released at the level of the myotendinous junction, then strongly pulled and transferred intra-articularly through two 8 mm transtibial and transfemoral tunnels emerging just in the sites of origin and the insertion site of the native ACL (Fig. 1.5).

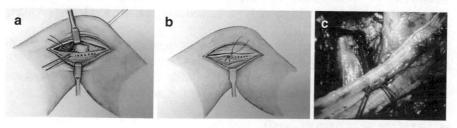

Fig. 1.2 (**a**, **b**) Andrews technique with transosseous sutures, as reported in the "Atlante di Chirurgia Ortopedica" by L. Perugia, G. Puddu, PP. Mariani, A. Ferretti in 1985 (Courtesy of Biagio Moretti; reprinted with permission). (**c**) Intraoperative findings of the same technique

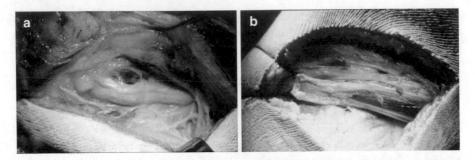

Fig. 1.3 (**a, b**) Identification of the peroneal nerve required for the advancement of the biceps tendon. (**b**) Advancement of the biceps tendon according to Hughston

Fig. 1.4 Advancement of the POL and semimembranosus tendon according to Hughston

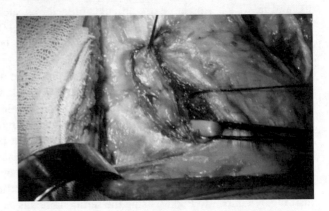

The anatomy of the femoral origin of the ACL was reproduced thanks to an original offset guide (Fig. 1.6).

The guide, once anchored behind the femoral condyle, allowed us to drill the femoral tunnel from the outside-in, emerging just in front of the over-the-top position at the level of ACL origin. The bone plug in the femoral tunnel provided bone-to-bone healing, which was also ensured by postoperative immobilization in flexion for several weeks (4–6 weeks).

One of the main advantages of this technique relied on the preservation of the flexion and the internal rotation strength of the hamstrings, as shown by an isokinetic dynamometric evaluation study performed using the first available isokinetic dynamometer, Cybex II [15].

In most severe cases and high-risk patients, the procedure was associated with extra-articular tenodesis to better control rotational instability and pivot shift.

The principles of the technique proposed by Puddu and strongly supported by the chief of our department, Professor Lamberto Perugia, are as follows:

– Use of the hamstrings as a graft.
– Careful regard of the anatomy of the ACL through outside-in femoral drilling.
– Extra-articular reconstruction as an additional procedure in selected cases.

Fig. 1.5 ACL reconstruction with semitendinosus and gracilis tendons according to the technique originally described by Puddu G (reprinted with permission from "Atlante di Chirurgia Ortopedica Vol.II" Bari 1985, courtesy of Biagio Moretti) [8]

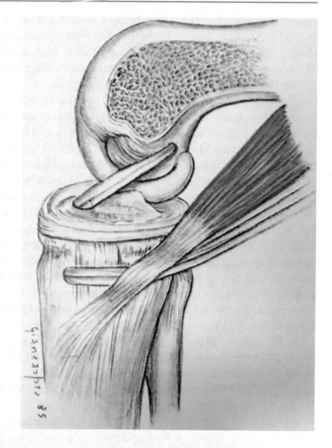

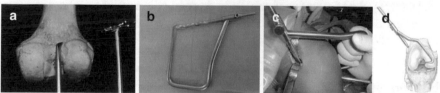

Fig. 1.6 Puddu's offset guide allowed the femoral tunnel to emerge in the insertion site of the native ACL, just in front of the top position. (**a, c, d**) placement of the tip of the guide in the over-the-top position; (**b**) the offset guide. (**d**): reprinted with permission from Citieffe catalogue (Bologna, Italy)

These three principles represent the basis of our philosophy of treatment for ACL-deficient knees, and they remain unchanged to date, even if several changes have occurred in surgical techniques (from open to arthroscopic-assisted), fixation devices, harvesting techniques and postoperative courses and rehabilitation.

The original Puddu technique has been used for several years, especially for athletes, including professional football players. I had the chance to personally follow up many of them in long postoperative rehabilitation, which lasted up to 10 months before return to the sport was eventually allowed. I will never forget the case of one of the most important players of the AS Roma, Carlo Ancelotti, who was treated with this technique for both knees over a period of 3 years and returned to play at the preinjury level (Serie A and Italian National Team). During the 1990 FIFA World Cup, when I made my debut as the team physician on the bench of the Italian National Team, Carlo was still in the game.

The Puddu technique was later given up, mainly due to postoperative pain, prolonged immobilization and long, stressful and exhaustive rehabilitation, which resulted in a delayed return to daily life activities and sport performance.

However, even when the technique was modified (use of the arthroscopy-assisted technique, proximal tendon detachment, the use of a free graft, lateral tenodesis techniques and accelerated rehabilitation), the principles that inspired the original technique remained unchanged. Thanks to this unshakable confidence in our principles, we continued using the hamstrings as the graft of choice, respecting the original ACL anatomy by drilling the femoral tunnel from the outside to the inside, and using extra-articular reconstruction whenever needed. This attitude did not change even when, in the nineties and in the first decade of the twenty-first century, a single-incision vertically placed bone-patellar-tendon-bone (BPTB) graft (the Rosenberg technique) [16] was considered the gold standard for ACL reconstruction worldwide. The remarkable and probably unique experience we obtained during these years has given us the opportunity to authoritatively argue with all international experts.

In this context, all the studies published by our group over the last decades should be credited [1, 17–26]; not only because they deal with medium- and long-term results but also because they analyse all aspects of the procedures: the biomechanics of the graft and the fixation devices; tendon regeneration and its consequences on flexion mechanism; and any possible complications.

Currently, as most surgeons around the world have reconsidered the use of the hamstrings [27], as well as the importance of reproducing the anatomy of the original ACL [21], the advantages of outside-in femoral drilling [26] and the significant role of extra-articular reconstruction [28], we are very proud of our original and steady choice.

References

1. Ferretti A. A historical note on anterior cruciate ligament reconstruction. JBJS. 2003;85:970–1.
2. Galeazzi R. La ricostituzione dei legamenti crociati del ginocchio. Atti e Memorie della Società Lombarda di Chirurgia. 1934;II:302–16.
3. Jones R, Smith SA. On rupture of the crucial ligaments of the knee and on fractures of the spine of the tibia. Br J Surg. 1913;1:70–89.
4. Slocum DB, Larson RL. Rotatory instability of the knee. Its pathogenesis and a clinical test to demonstrate its presence. J Bone Joint Surg Am. 1968;50(2):211–25.
5. Torg JS, Conrad W, Kalen V. Clinical diagnosis of anterior cruciate ligament instability in the athlete. Am J Sports Med. 1976;4(2):84–93.
6. Galway R, Beaupre A, MacIntosh D. Pivot shift: a clinical sign of symptomatic anterior cruciate insufficiency. J Bone Joint Surg Br. 1972;54:763–4.
7. Hughston JC, Andrews JR, Cross MJ, Moschi A. Classification of knee ligament instabilities. Part I. The medial compartment and cruciate ligaments. J Bone Joint Surg Am. 1976;58(2):159–72.

8. Puddu G. Method for reconstruction of the anterior cruciate ligament using the semitendinosus tendon. Am J Sports Med. 1980; PMID: 7435756
9. Norwood LA. Treatment of acute anterolateral rotatory instability. Orthop Clin North Am. 1985;16(1):127–34.
10. Norwood LA Jr, Hughston JC. 1. Combined anterolateral-anteromedial rotatory instability of the knee. Clin Orthop Relat Res. 1980;147:62–7.
11. Terry GC, Hughston JC, Norwood LA. 1. The anatomy of the iliopatellar band and iliotibial tract. Am J Sports Med. 1986;14(1):39–45.
12. Feagin JA. The crucial ligaments. New York: Churchill Livingstone; 1988.
13. Müller W. (transl. Tegler TG). The knee: form, function, and ligament reconstruction. Springer-Verlag; 1983.
14. Perugia L, Puddu G, Mariani PP, Ferretti A. Chronic anteromedial and anterolateral instability of the knee in athletes. Results of treatment with peripheral surgery. Rev Chir Orthop Reparatrice Appar Mot. 1982;68(6):365–8.
15. Mariani PP, Ferretti A, Gigli C, Puddu G. Isokinetic evaluation of the knee after arthroscopic meniscectomy: comparison between anterolateral and central approaches. Arthroscopy. 1987;3(2):123–6.
16. Rosenberg TD. Technique for endoscopic method of ACL reconstruction. Norwood, MA: Microsurgical, Inc; 1989.
17. Ferretti A, De Carli A, Conteduca F, Mariani PP, Fontana M. The results of reconstruction of the anterior cruciate ligament with semitendinosus and gracilis tendons in chronic laxity of the knee. Ital J Orthop Traumatol. 1989;15(4):415–24.
18. Ferretti A, Conteduca F, De Carli A, Fontana M, Mariani PP. Results of reconstruction of the anterior cruciate ligament with the tendons of semitendinosus and gracilis in acute capsulo-ligamentous lesions of the knee. Ital J Orthop Traumatol. 1990;16(4):452–8.
19. Ferretti A, Papandrea P, Conteduca F, Mariani PP. Knee ligament injuries in volleyball players. Am J Sports Med. 1992;20(2):203–7.
20. Ferretti A, Conteduca F, Labianca L., Monaco E, De Carli A. Evolgate fixation of doubled flexor graft in anterior cruciate ligament reconstruction: biomechanical evaluation with cyclic loading. Am J Sports Med. 2005;33(4):574–82.
21. Ferretti A, Monaco E, Ponzo A, Basiglini L, Iorio R, Caperna L, Conteduca F. Combined intra-articular and extra-articular reconstruction in anterior cruciate ligament-deficient knee: 25 years later. Arthroscopy. 2016;32(10):2039–47.
22. Ferretti A, Monaco E, Ponzo A, Dagget M, Guzzini M, Mazza D, et al. The unhappy triad of the knee re-revisited. Int Orthop. 2019;43(1):223–8.
23. Guzzini M, Mazza D, Fabbri M, Lanzetti R, Redler A, Iorio C, et al. Extra-articular tenodesis combined with an anterior cruciate ligament reconstruction in acute anterior cruciate ligament tear in elite female football players. Int Orthop. 2016;40(10):2091–6.
24. Iorio R, Vadalà A, Di Vavo I, De Carli A, Conteduca F, Argento G, Ferretti A. Tunnel enlargement after anterior cruciate ligament reconstruction in patients with post-operative septic arthritis. Knee Surg Sports Traumatol Arthrosc. 2008;16(10):921–7.
25. Monaco E, Labianca L, Speranza A, Agrò AM, Camillieri G, D'Arrigo C, Ferretti A. Biomechanical evaluation of different anterior cruciate ligament fixation techniques for hamstring graft. J Orthop Sci. 2010;15(1):125–31.
26. Monaco E, Fabbri M, Redler A, Iorio R, Conteduca J, Argento G, Ferretti A. In-out versus out-in technique for ACL reconstruction: a prospective clinical and radiological comparison. J Orthop Traumatol. 2017;18(4):335–41.
27. Thaunat M, Fayard JM, Sonnery-Cottet B. Hamstring tendons or bone-patellar tendon-bone graft for anterior cruciate ligament reconstruction? Orthop Traumatol Surg Res. 2019;105(1S):S89–94.
28. Tramer JS, Fidai MS, Kadri O, et al. Anterolateral ligament reconstruction practice patterns across the United States. Orthop J Sports Med. 2018;6(12):2325967118811063.

Anatomy of Secondary Restraints of ACL

Andrea Ferretti, Matteo Guzzini, and Edoardo Viglietta

The knee is the joint of the lower limb, located between the hip and the ankle; among the weight-bearing joints, it has the lowest degree of geometrical congruence, resulting in the lowest level of intrinsic stability.

Unlike other joints, the knee does not include any mechanical interlock between its articular surfaces. While in the hip, the femoral head deeply recesses into the acetabular cup and in the ankle, the talus stands into the malleolar pinch, in the knee, the cylindrical femoral condyles lie over the quite flat surface of the tibial plateau (Fig. 2.1).

Joint stability is a crucial factor in most daily life activities, such as maintaining the standing position and walking, running, and jumping; due to a lack of any mechanical constraints, knee stability is almost exclusively provided by ligaments, which have a very complex functional anatomy.

Knee ligaments can be divided into three compartments:

- The medial compartment medially extends from the patellar tendon to the tibial insertion of the posterior cruciate ligament (PCL).
- The lateral compartment laterally extends from the patellar tendon to the tibial insertion of the PCL.
- The central pivot is composed of two cruciate ligaments.

While Hughston et al. [1, 2] defined anterolateral rotatory instability (ALRI) as primarily resulting from a tear of the middle third of the lateral capsular ligament accentuated by a tear of the anterior cruciate ligament (ACL), later, most

A. Ferretti (✉) · M. Guzzini · E. Viglietta
Orthopaedic Unit, Sant'Andrea University Hospital, La Sapienza University, Rome, Italy

© The Author(s), under exclusive license to Springer Nature Switzerland AG 2022
A. Ferretti (ed.), *Anterolateral Rotatory Instability in ACL Deficient Knee*, https://doi.org/10.1007/978-3-031-00115-4_2

11

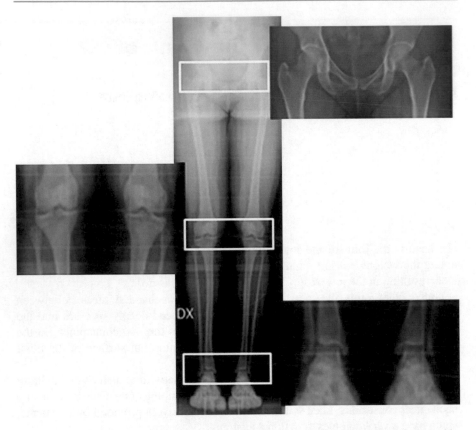

Fig. 2.1 Weight-bearing X-rays of the lower limbs showing the different congruence between hip, knee, and ankle joints

researchers described ALRI and the pivot shift phenomenon as the result of an anterior cruciate ligament (ACL) injury eventually associated with a secondary restraint lesion, which significantly affects the severity of the instability. Therefore, as this pattern of knee instability is strictly related to injuries of the ACL and secondary restraints of the lateral compartment, a detailed description of these structures is essential. Surprisingly, even the anatomy of this area is still a matter of great debate.

The anterior portion of the external compartment is made up of a tiny layer of capsule that is slightly enforced by the extensions of the quadriceps tendon and seems to be biomechanically ineffective; it is the medial third, which appears to be the most important structure because of its role in controlling the internal rotation of the tibia [1, 2].

In the late nineteenth century, a French doctor, Paul Segond, was the first to report the existence of a thick ligamentous structure in the external compartment of the knee, which could play a role in controlling tibial internal rotation. In the well-known paper "Recherches Cliniques Et Expérimentales Sur Les Épanchements Sanguins Du Genou Par Entorse" (knee haemarthrosis as a result of ligament sprains) [3], the author reported a resistant, pearly coloured fibrous tissue band, which was stretched during varus-internal rotation stress. This band was strong enough to be able to tear off its bone insertion in case of avulsion. This avulsion fracture is still known as a "Segond's fracture"; it is considered an indirect radiological sign of an ACL injury and is often associated with it (Fig. 2.2).

In the last century, many authors have studied anterolateral compartment anatomy, but the results have often been conflicting.

J. Hughston et al. [1, 2], in their well-known studies in which Segond's fracture was never mentioned, described the anterolateral capsular ligament's medial third as capsular thickening; this structure was crucial in supporting the ACL in controlling tibial internal rotation: as a consequence, whenever this ligament is injured, there will be a rotatory instability (detectable by the "jerk test").

Later, Feagin's observations were roughly the same. In his book "The Crucial Ligaments" [4], he refers to Segond's fracture and describes a clear thickening in the joint capsule at the anterolateral level, clearly suggesting the existence of a real capsular ligament (Fig. 2.3).

Unlike the other authors, Werner Müller [5] had different conclusions. In his masterpiece "The Knee: Form, Function, and Ligament Reconstruction", he also identified rotatory instability resulting from a combined injury of the ACL and anterolateral peripheral structures. However, he identified and described the anterolateral femorotibial ligament (ALFTL) as a part of the fascia lata. More specifically,

Fig. 2.2 Segond's fracture: an avulsion fracture of the lateral tibial plateau

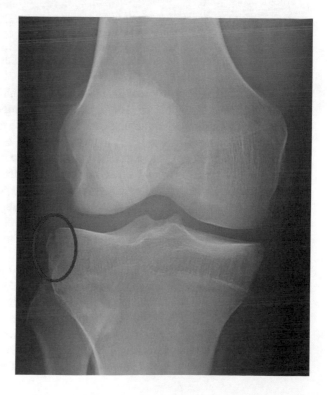

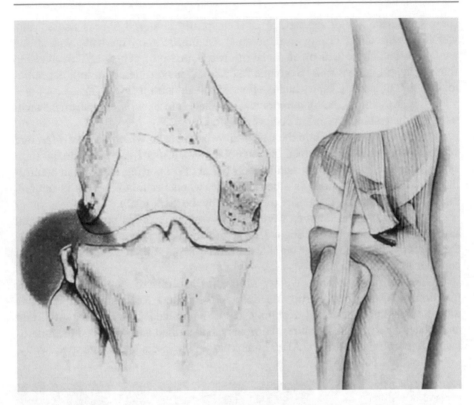

Fig. 2.3 Pathogenesis of Segond's fracture as reported by Feagin et al. in "The Crucial Ligaments" on pages 51 and 54. Churchill Livingstone, 1988 [4]. Reprinted with permission

it was the deep posterior portion of the iliotibial tract, which is attached to the inter-muscular septum proximal to the lateral collateral ligament (LCL) on the femoral condyle (Kaplan fibres), that, running over the joint line towards Gerdy's tubercle, acts as a true ligament. Unlike the structures identified by Segond, Hughston, and Feagin, Müller did not refer to a capsular ligament, as the ALFTL he identified actu-ally runs in a more superficial layer bridging the joint and the capsule itself. However, later in his book, Müller recognized that in the posterior half of the lateral capsule, a stronger femorotibial structure exists, with the avulsion fragment described by Segond on the lateral tibial plateau just below the articular cartilage and above the fibular head as proof of the existence of tension-resistant collagenous fibres in the lateral capsule.

The complex anatomy of the iliotibial tract was also thoroughly investigated by some Hughston's fellows. Among them, Terry et al., in their work "The anatomy of the iliopatellar band and iliotibial tract" [6], identified the capsulo-osseous layer as an expansion of the iliotibial tract originating from the intermuscular septum and inserting into the lateral capsule and the tibia just posterior to Gerdy's tubercle, sug-gesting its role as a true anterolateral ligament of the knee. In a further study [7] based on surgical findings, the same authors reported how injuries of the deep capsulo-osseous layers often occur along with ACL tears. They also suggested a sort of synergism between these structures that could form a sling behind the lateral femoral condyle, preventing the pivot shift phenomenon (inverted U or horseshoe effect: Fig. 2.4).

In 2013, Claes et al. [9] published a very detailed anatomical study of a true capsular ligament, the anterolateral ligament (ALL), carefully describing its insertions and course, and in a later study [10], its morphological and biomechanical characteristics. Claes' studies had a great mediatic impact, as the scientific community was surprised to hear that a new knee ligament was discovered in the twenty-first century.

Based on dissections performed on 41 cadaver knees, the authors were able to identify a well-defined ligamentous structure that was clearly distinguishable from the anterolateral capsule in all but one specimen. This anterolateral ligament originated close to the lateral femoral epicondyle slightly anterior to the origin of the lateral collateral ligament (LCL); it showed an oblique course to the anterolateral aspect of the proximal tibia with firm attachment to the lateral meniscus, thus

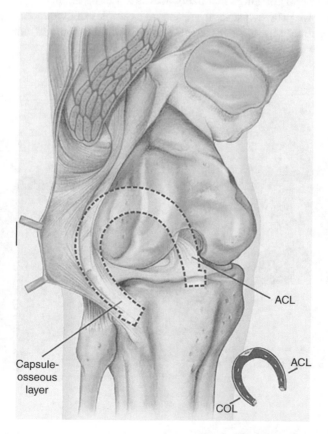

Fig. 2.4 The horseshoe effect, formed by the capsulo-osseous layer of the iliotibial tract and the ACL, resulting in an inverted "U" (reprinted with permission from Viera et al.) [8]

enveloping the inferior lateral geniculate artery and vein. Its insertion was grossly located midway between Gerdy's tubercle and the tip of fibular head, definitively separated from the iliotibial band. The mean length of the ALL was 41 mm in flexion and 38 mm in extension, with a mean width of approximately 10 mm and a thickness at the joint line of 1 mm. During manipulation of the knee, maximal tension of the ligament was observed in mid-flexion and during internal rotation of the tibia (Fig. 2.5).

The work of Claes et al. was widely debated, as many authors disagreed with their findings. The main question raised was whether the existence of the ALL was a myth or reality [9, 11].

However, Claes and coauthors should be credited for refocusing attention on the secondary restraints of the ACL, which were forgotten by most surgeons worldwide. In fact, since the Claes report, many other papers on this subject have been published, most of them supporting their findings [12–14].

Personally, we believe there is no doubt regarding the existence of an anatomical anterolateral capsular reinforcement corresponding to the structure brilliantly illustrated by Claes and coauthors that likely acts as a true ligament.

In support, we provided several substantial examples of evidence.

Following the dissection methods proposed by Claes, some of our fellows carried out further anatomical studies.

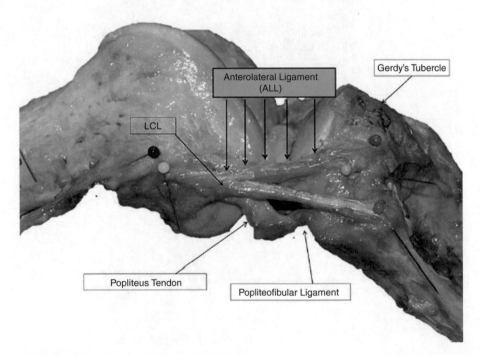

Fig. 2.5 Anatomy of the anterolateral ligament as reported by Claes et al. (9) (reprinted with permission)

Daggett et al. [12], in their cadaveric dissection study, clearly described the steps to identify the anterolateral ligament of the knee: "*The ALL can be easily identified and isolated through meticulous dissection in three steps: (1) Iliotibial band reflection is performed in a proximal-to-distal direction with preservation of the structures deep to the iliotibial band. (2) The ALL is identified by flexing the knee between 30° and 60° and applying an internal rotation force. This is followed by posterior capsulectomy through reflection of the biceps femoris, isolation of the lateral collateral ligament, and removal of the capsule between the posterior boundary of the ALL and lateral collateral ligament. (3) Anterior capsulectomy is performed through the removal of all anterior tissues bordering the anterior boundary of the ALL*".

As the same authors state in their conclusion: "*The ALL exists as a distinct, extra-articular lateral structure of the knee. The origin of the ALL is bony in nature, with an attachment slightly posterior and proximal to the lateral femoral epicondyle. The ALL also has some fibres attached to the lateral meniscus, with the main insertion attaching onto the tibia between the Gerdy tubercle and the fibular head*".

More evidence of the exact nature of the ALL was provided by Redler et al. [15] in their microscopic and ultrastructural study. Eight samples of the ALL, anterolateral capsule, and medial collateral ligament (MCL) harvested from 4 fresh-frozen specimens were evaluated by light microscopy, variable pressure-scanning pressure microscopy, and transmission electron microscopy. By analysing the structure and ultrastructure of the ALL (Figs. 2.6 and 2.7) compared to the other knee ligaments and capsules, they confirmed the ligamentous structure of the ALL. They stated that "Ultrastructure *analysis demonstrated similar morphology between the ALL and MCL, with significant differences in these two structures compared with the joint*

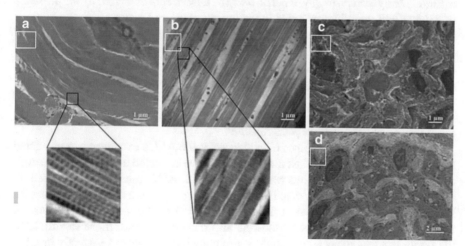

Fig. 2.6 Ultrastructural morphology of the ALL, MCL, and joint capsule. (**a**) ALL collagen and (**b**) MCL collagen fibres. Insets: identically sized magnified areas of aligned fibrils of the corresponding figures. (**c**) Anterolateral capsule surrounding the ALL. (**d**) Synovial cells of the joint capsule. *ALL* anterolateral ligament, *MCL* medial collateral ligament (modified from Redler et al. [15])

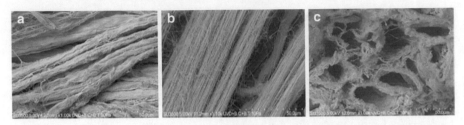

Fig. 2.7 Three-dimensional surface morphology of the ALL, MCL, and joint capsule. (**a**) ALL and (**b**) MCL bundle fibres. (**c**) Microcavities of the joint capsule surrounding the ALL. *ALL* anterolateral ligament, *MCL* medial collateral ligament (modified from Redler et al. [15])

Fig. 2.8 Surgical finding of a Segond's fracture

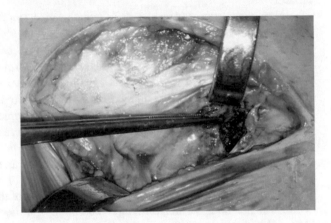

capsule. On light microscopy, the ALL and MCL were characterized by the presence of a dense collagen fibre oriented in the longitudinal and transversal directions of the fibre bundles, while the joint capsule was found to have a more disorganized architecture. On transmission electron microscopy, the collagen fibres of the ALL and MCL demonstrated similar ultrastructural morphology, with both having collagen fibres in parallel, longitudinal alignment... Variable pressure-scanning electron microscopy highlighted that ALL and MCL morphology demonstrated arrangements of fibre bundles that are densely packed and organized, in contrast to the disorganized fibres of the joint capsule".

Another very important piece of evidence for the ALL's existence is represented by Segond's fracture. In the last few years, we have collected a large series of surgically treated Segond's fractures where refixation of the fragment was performed. In all cases, the fracture was detected at a tibial level, deep down the fascia lata and the iliotibial tract, just at the site of the distal insertion of the anterolateral ligament, about halfway between Gerdy's tubercle and the fibular head. More superficially, the fascia lata was intact or just slightly stretched but was always perfectly inserted into Gerdy's tubercle. With regard to the bone fragment, it was clear that only the joint capsule was attached to it (Fig. 2.8).

As only a strong ligament or a ligamentous structure can be responsible for an avulsion fracture in case of extreme traction, it currently seems anachronistic and illogic to deny the existence of the ALL or an ALL-like structure.

An interesting question is whether the ALL can be considered a single structure that is able to act as the only secondary restraint of the ACL in controlling the rotatory stability and pivot shift phenomenon, or is a part of a series of structures that synergically carry out the same function.

As far as we are concerned, and in agreement with others, we consider the ALL as the main structure of a group of structures (the anterolateral complex), that also includes the deep portion of the iliotibial tract (capsulo-osseous layer as described by Terry et al. [7]) and the posterior horn of the lateral meniscus. The primary role attributed to the ALL is related to the high prevalence of its injuries occurring along with ACL tears and to their biomechanical effects as the main factor responsible for an explosive pivot shift (+++) [16, 17].

Amazingly enough, it could be beneficial to reconsider the anatomical features as presented by J. Hughston et al. in their 1976 works [1, 2]. While examining the anatomy of the medial and lateral compartments, the authors realized how both compartments seem to disclose a similar feature. In the medial compartment, they identified a superficial and a deep medial collateral ligament. The superficial layer (the "medial collateral ligament", as commonly described in anatomy books), which has a ribbon-like shape, originates from the medial femoral epicondyle, and then inserts down to the tibia deeply to the pes anserinus tendons. The ligament bridges the capsule being separated from it by a deep bursa. The deep layer is actually a reinforcement of the capsule or a capsular ligament, which is divided into two parts: the longer, proximal, meniscofemoral ligament and the shorter, distal, meniscotibial ligament, both of which are firmly attached to the medial meniscus.

The same architecture could be identified in the lateral compartment. The superficial layer would be represented by the deep part of the iliotibial tract, which originates from the lateral femoral epicondyle, bridges the joint and inserts itself into Gerdy's tubercle, running almost parallel to the MCL (Fig. 2.9). The deep layer, represented by the "medial third of the anterolateral capsular ligament" (currently called the "ALL"), could, in turn, be divided into meniscofemoral and meniscotibial parts.

In fact, in our dissections, as well as in the original description by Claes, the ALL has tight connections with the lateral meniscus (Fig. 2.10). Moreover, Corbo et al. [18], in a histological and biomechanical study on the ALL, recognized the two components of the ALL (superior meniscofemoral and inferior meniscotibial), also showing that the infra-meniscal fibres were stronger and stiffer than the supra-meniscal fibres.

This appealing description might help surgeons to better understand the complex anatomy of the anterolateral compartment of the knee, whose role in maintaining rotational stability should no longer be questioned.

Fig. 2.9 The anterolateral femoral tibial ligament, as described by Muller, runs almost parallel to the medial collateral ligament and possibly acts as a superficial layer of the ALL (modified from "Muller W. The Knee: Form, Function, and Ligament Reconstruction, 1982 [5]")

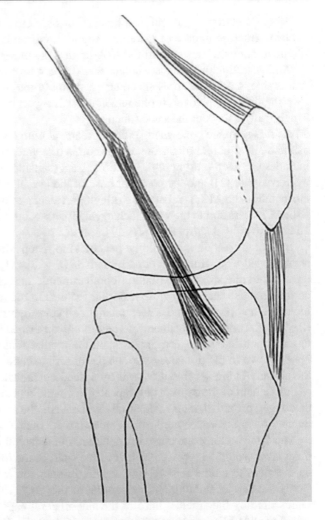

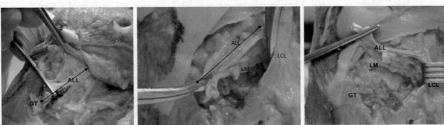

Fig. 2.10 Dissection of the anterolateral compartment of the knee. Note the connection between the ALL detached from Gerdy's tubercle and the peripheral rim of the lateral meniscus (C). GT: Gerdy's Tubercle, LCL: Lateral Collateral Ligament, LM: Lateral Meniscus

References

1. Hughston JC, Andrews JR, Cross MJ, et al. Classification of knee ligament instabilities. Part I. The medial compartment and cruciate ligaments. J Bone Jt Surg. American volume. 1976;58(2):159–72.
2. Hughston JC, Andrews JR, Cross MJ, et al. Classification of knee ligament instabilities. Part II. The lateral compartment. J Bone J Surg. American volume. 1976;58(2):173–9.
3. Segond PF. Recherches Cliniques Et Expérimentales Sur Les Épanchements Sanguins Du Genou Par Entorse. 1879.
4. Feagin JA. The Crucial Ligaments. Churchill Livingstone; 1988.
5. Muller W. The Knee, form, function, and ligament reconstruction. Springer Verlag; 1982.
6. Terry GC, Hughston JC, Norwood LA. The anatomy of the iliopatellar band and iliotibial tract. Am J Sports Med. 1986;14(1):39–45.
7. Terry GC, Norwood LA, Hughston JC, Caldwell KM. How iliotibial tract injuries of the knee combine with acute anterior cruciate ligament tears to influence abnormal anterior tibial displacement. Am J Sports Med. 1993;21(1):55–60.
8. Vieira EL, Vieira EA, Da Silva RT, Berlfein PA, Abdalla RJ, Cohen M. An anatomic study of the iliotibial tract. Arthroscopy. 2007;23:269–74.
9. Claes S, Vereecke E, Maes M, Victor J, Verdonk P, Bellemans J. Anatomy of the anterolateral ligament of the knee. Journal of anatomy. 2013;223(4):321–8.
10. Claes S, Luyckx T, Vereecke E, Bellemans J. The Segond fracture: a bony injury of the anterolateral ligament of the knee. Arthroscopy. 2014;30(11):1475–82.
11. Musahl V, Rahnemai-Azar AA, Van Eck CF, Guenther D, Fu FH. Anterolateral ligament of the knee, fact or fiction? Knee Surg Sports Traumatol Arthrosc. 2016;24(1):2–3.
12. Daggett M, Busch K, Sonnery-Cottet B. Surgical dissection of the anterolateral ligament. Arthrosc Tech. 2016;5(1):e185–8.
13. Helito CP, Demange MK, Bonadio MB, Tírico LE, Gobbi RG, Pécora JR, Camanho GL. Anatomy and Histology of the Knee Anterolateral Ligament. Orthop J Sports Med. 2013;1(7):2325967113513546.
14. Sonnery-Cottet B, Lutz C, Daggett M, Dalmay F, Freychet B, Niglis L, et al. The involvement of the anterolateral ligament in rotational control of the knee. Am J Sports Med. 2016;44:1209–14.
15. Redler A, Miglietta S, Monaco E, Matassa R, Relucenti M, Daggett M, Ferretti A, Familiari G. Ultrastructural assessment of the anterolateral ligament. Orthop J Sports Med. 2019;7(12):2325967119887920.
16. Ferretti A, Monaco E, Fabbri M, Maestri B, De Carli A. Prevalence and classification of injuries of anterolateral complex in acute anterior cruciate ligament tears. Arthroscopy. 2017;33(1):147–54.
17. Ferretti A, Monaco E, Gaj E, Andreozzi V, Annibaldi A, Carrozzo A, Vieira TD, Sonnery-Cottet B, Saithna A. Risk factors for Grade 3 pivot shift in knees with acute anterior cruciate ligament injuries: a comprehensive evaluation of the importance of osseous and soft tissue parameters from the SANTI Study Group. Am J Sports Med. 2020;48(10):2408–17.
18. Corbo G, Norris M, Getgood A, Burkhart TA. The infra-meniscal fibers of the anterolateral ligament are stronger and stiffer than the supra-meniscal fibers despite similar histological characteristics. Knee Surg Sports Traumatol Arthrosc. 2017;25(4):1078–85.

Biomechanics of Anterolateral Instability and Pivot Shift

3

Andrea Ferretti and Susanna M. Pagnotta

Since the first description of the pivot shift phenomenon and the recognition of anterolateral instability in ACL-deficient knees, researchers and surgeons have focused on the pathogenesis and biomechanics of this intriguing aspect of knee surgery. In fact, since the seventies and eighties, most authors agreed that even if the pivot shift phenomenon was related to ACL insufficiency, it was severely increased by tears of the secondary restraints of the lateral compartment [1]. Hughston and other famous knee surgeons considered isolated ACL lesions to be extremely rare, if not impossible; they postulated that the injury responsible for a change in the biomechanics of the knee was that of the secondary restraints. With the advent of arthroscopy, however, the interest of surgeons shifted towards intra-articular structures, which are easily investigated by the scope, and the possible role of extra-articular structures, well recognized and defined previously, was almost completely neglected [2–4].

Our interest in the biomechanics of anterolateral rotatory instability of the knee has been stimulated by the advent of surgical navigation systems in our hospital. We have performed some studies in this field, in some ways unique in their kind, which deserve to be described in detail, as they provide a substantial contribution to the understanding of this issue.

The aim of the first study [5], published in the KSSTA in 2012, was to evaluate the kinematic changes occurring in the knee after a lesion of the ACL, whether combined with an anterolateral capsular ligament lesion. This study was published 2 years before the anatomical study of Claes et al.[6] and a similar biomechanical study by the same authors on this topic, which received an award from the European Society of Sports Traumatology, Knee Surgery and Arthroscopy (ESSKA) [7].

A. Ferretti (✉) · S. M. Pagnotta
Orthopaedic Unit, Sant'Andrea University Hospital, La Sapienza University, Rome, Italy

A. Ferretti (ed.), *Anterolateral Rotatory Instability in ACL Deficient Knee*,
https://doi.org/10.1007/978-3-031-00115-4_3

23

The null hypothesis of our study was that not all ACL lesions result in the same degree of joint laxity. Compared to similar studies with cadavers, which analysed amputated knees, the advantage of our study was that we used the entire lower limb with all muscle insertions and the periarticular tissues intact [8–10]. Another important characteristic of our study was the use of the surgical navigation system for biomechanical analyses. The main advantage of the studies performed with the aid of a navigation system, compared to the robot-like devices used by others [9], in which the pivot shift phenomenon is only simulated, consists of the chance to accurately replicate any possible test, including a real pivot shift test. The reliability of the navigation has been previously tested [11], and the extreme precision of the system to detect even minor displacement between the tibia and the femur in three dimensions, with errors of 1 mm and 1°, is widely recognized. Considering the reliability of this technique and the integrity of the periarticular tissues, this study would be regarded as more accurate and reliable than other cadaveric studies in which the overall stability of the knee could be compromised as a result of amputation: The lack of integrity of important knee stabilizers such as the biceps femoris, the fascia lata and the semimembranosus could jeopardize the overall stability of the knee and the effect of further cutting procedures.

In our study, we evaluated 10 lower limbs with intact knees without a history or the appearance of previous pathologies. A 2.0 OrthoPilot ACL navigation system (B. Braun Aesculap, Tuttlingen, Germany) was used to calculate the knee kinematics. This system measured the anterior tibial translation (ATT), internal rotation (IR), and external rotation (ER) of the tibia in relation to the femur. The femoral and tibial transmitters were attached using 2.5-mm K-wires. Different extra-articular landmarks were entered into the system using the straight pointer (third transmitter) (Fig. 3.1).

Knee flexion and external and internal rotation were also performed to calibrate the system. The kinematics were evaluated under the following conditions: with all the structures intact; after cutting the PL bundle of the ACL (performed arthroscopically with shavers and scissors); complete arthroscopic lesion of both the PL and AM bundles of the ACL; and after the lesion of the anterolateral portion of the knee joint capsule. The anterolateral aspect of the knee was approached through a hockey stick skin incision, the iliotibial tract was divided along its fibres, and the articular

Fig. 3.1 Knee transmitters fixed to bones for navigation

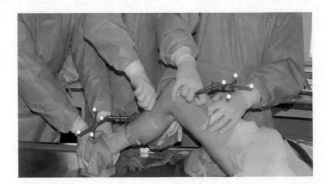

Fig. 3.2 Tear of the anterolateral capsule

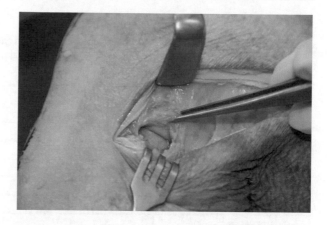

capsule was exposed. An incision approximately 2 cm long was made through the anterolateral ligament (ALL) at the level of the lateral joint line, below the lateral meniscus, in a region often found injured in vivo (Fig. 3.2). In each of the four phases of the procedure, the following measurements were made: the maximal anterior translation of the tibia on the femur at 30°, 60° and 90° of knee flexion and the maximal IR and ER of the tibia at 0°, 15°, 30°, 45°, 60° and 90° of flexion. Moreover, the same senior surgeon clinically evaluated the knee using the Lachman test (evaluated as positive or negative) and the pivot shift test (evaluated 1+ as a glide, 2+ as a clunk and 3+ as a subluxation).

The first important result of this study was that cutting the PL bundle alone (real partial lesion of the ligament) did not result in any detectable change in either the anterior translation or rotatory stability. A significant increase in anterior tibial translation (in all degrees of flexion) was observed only after complete resection of the two bundles of the ACL. The anterior translation of the tibia was further increased by the anterolateral capsular lesion only at 60° of flexion (Table 3.1).

Concerning rotation, neither partial (PL) nor complete (PL+AM) ACL lesions resulted in a statistically significant change, while the combined lesion of the anterolateral capsule (AL capsule) produced a rotatory instability that was statistically significant at 30°, 45°, 60° and 90° of flexion (Table 3.2).

Clinically, the Lachman test became positive only after the complete ACL lesion and persisted after the combined AL capsule lesion. The effect of the sequential cuts on the pivot shift test was even more interesting and less predictable. The test remained negative after the isolated PL lesion; after the complete ACL lesion, the pivot shift test continued to be undetectable in two cases, mild (grade 1+) in seven cases and moderate (grade 2+) in only one case. The additional lesion of the AL capsule resulted in an increase in the pivot shift grade in all cases, with a pivot shift grade of 2+ in 3 cadavers and a grade of 3+ in the other 7 cadavers (Table 3.3).

The most important finding of this study was that our hypothesis was confirmed; an ACL lesion can result in different degrees of instability; an isolated ACL lesion is not always able to produce biomechanically relevant and clinically detectable rotatory instability, while an associated lesion of the AL capsule significantly

Table 3.1 Antero-posterior tibial translation at different degrees of knee flexion

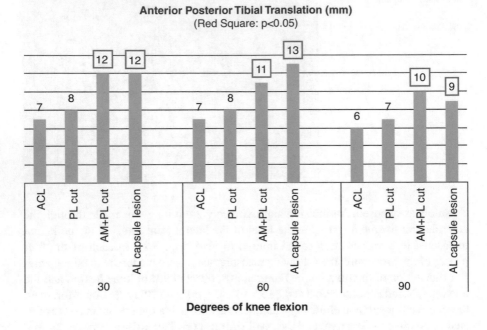

Table 3.2 Complete knee rotation at different degrees of knee flexion

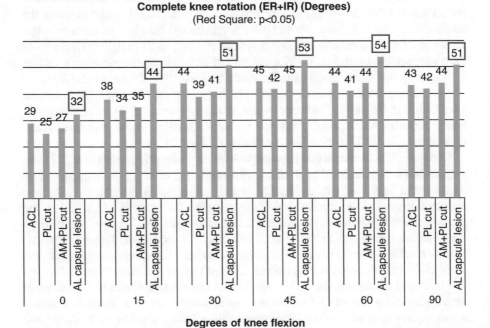

Table 3.3 The effect of sequential cuts on the pivot shift test

	Pivot shift test
Intact Knee	−10/10
PL cut	−10/10
AM + PL cut (ACL tear)	−2/10
	+7/10
	++1/10
ACL tear + AL capsule cut	−0/10
	+0/10
	++3/10
	+++7/10

PL Posterolateral bundle of the ACL; *AM* Antero Medial bundle; *AL* Antero Lateral

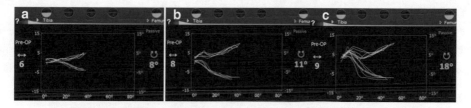

Fig. 3.3 Navigation system charts (**a**) before cutting, (**b**) ACL deficient, (**c**) ACL + ALL deficient (yellow: indicates anterior tibial translation; Green: indicates tibial rotation)

increases rotatory instability. An isolated ACL lesion never results in a severe pivot shift grade (grade 3+), which can only be observed as a result of combined ACL and AL capsule lesions.

This study should be credited as it refocused the attention of knee surgeons on the role of the secondary restraints on the pathogenesis and biomechanics of antero-lateral rotatory instability (ALRI) and the pivot shift phenomenon at a time when the ACL seemed to be the only target of surgeons and researchers.

Almost 10 years after this publication, another in vivo study further validated these results [12, 13]. By analysing several anatomical and anatomo-surgical factors, including bone morphology and soft tissue injuries, in a consecutive series of 200 surgically treated acute ACL tears, the only factor that was statistically correlated with an explosive pivot shift phenomenon was eventual lesions of the antero-lateral ligament (ALL) [13].

The main limitation of our study was that the navigation system software only enabled us to perform static measurements of knee biomechanics, while a dynamic evaluation is required for a more precise assessment and measurement of the pivot shift test. The new OrthoPilot 2.2 navigation system allowed for a more accurate biomechanical investigation thanks to the ability of the software to record, with the same accuracy, the changes of the tibia on the femur occurring during dynamic tests and not just in static positions. The new software was not only able to record the anterior translation of the tibia during the Lachman test but also to analyse each component of the pivot shift test (translation and rotation) in all degrees of flexion and extension (Fig. 3.3).

Table 3.4 Mean anterior tibial translation (standard deviation) in millimetres, at 30° of flexion (Static Lachman test) for intact knee, ACL-deficient knee (ACL-D knee) and ACL and ALL-deficient knee (ACL+ALL-D knee). Red Square: $p < 0.05$

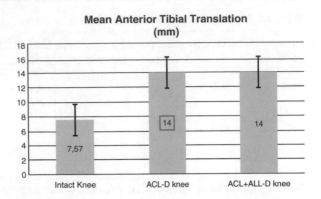

Similar to the previous work, we started with the hypothesis that an increased anterior translation of the tibia was a result of an isolated ACL lesion and the rotation of a combined lesion; the new software was used to record the tibial movements on the femur in 3 conditions: with intact ligaments, after an isolated complete ACL lesion and a combined ACL and ALL lesions. The procedure was the same as that described in the previous study, while dynamic measurements of ATT (anterior tibial translation) and ITR (internal tibial rotation) during the pivot shift test were performed for the intact knee, after cutting the isolated ACL lesion and after cutting the combined ACL and ALL lesions. The Lachman test and pivot shift test were performed by the same surgeon 3 times at each step, and the data were averaged by the navigation system. The pivot shift test was performed using manual loads applied by the same surgeon to minimize intra-observer variability. Again, in this study, entire lower limbs were used to maintain the periarticular structures and reproduce the correct clinical scenario.

The results confirmed the initial hypothesis of a statistically significant increase in the ATT during the Lachman test after complete resection of the ACL; this translation was not further increased after cutting the ALL (Table 3.4).

During the pivot shift test, a statistically significant increase in the ATT component was registered after cutting ACL with no further increase after ALL cutting. The ITR during the pivot shift was significantly increased both after cutting ACL and even more after ALL lesion (Table 3.5).

Overall, this study showed the difference between static and dynamic measurements occurring in the pivot shift test as a result of a torn ACL and its secondary restraints. Nevertheless, the results of the previous study were ultimately confirmed.

These results are in agreement with the findings of Parsons et al. [14] who reported that the ALL made a greater contribution to tibial internal rotation at higher degrees of flexion. However, this statement was based on an evaluation performed using a robotic testing system of the in situ forces acting on the ACL and ALL during the anterior drawer test and ITR (internal tibial rotation) separately. In a recent study, Bonanzinga et al. [15] used a different navigation system (Polaris; NDI,

Table 3.5 Mean Internal Tibial Rotation (standard deviation) in degrees, during pivot-shift test for intact knee, ACL-deficient knee (ACL-D knee) and ACL and ALL-deficient knee (ACL+ALL-D knee). Red Square: $p < 0.05$

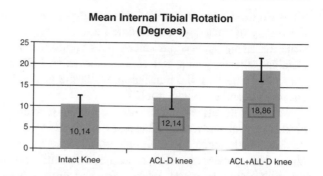

Waterloo, Ontario, Canada) to evaluate the effect of progressive lesions of the ACL and ALL during the pivot shift test. The laxity parameters evaluated during the pivot shift test were the acceleration displacement of the lateral tibial compartment and the amount of internal rotation. They found that although an isolated lesion of the ACL did not significantly affect acceleration, the ALL played a significant role in controlling acceleration during the pivot shift test. Similarly, Spencer et al. [16], in their sequential cutting study, found that the ALL was effective in controlling internal rotation in the setting of a combined complete ACL tear during the early phase of a simulated pivot shift test.

Other studies using different protocols led to the consideration of the iliotibial tract, instead of the ALL, as the main biomechanical factor in controlling internal rotation [17–19].

These studies had important potential biases related to the use of systems that only simulate clinical tests as well as the use of amputated knees with resected tendons and muscles. Moreover, by analysing the studies that emphasize the role of ITT from a clinical point of view, we should point out that injuries of the iliotibial tract seldom occur along with isolated ACL tears and are usually observed only in cases of more severe injuries and multiligamentous tears. Moreover, an iliotibial tract lesion would also affect and compromise the stability of the knee in the coronal plane, resulting in a positive varus test, which, on the contrary, is usually negative in any ALRI.

In conclusion, as a result of our experience and of our biomechanical studies, we can reasonably state the following:

(1) A partial tear of the ACL, limited to the PL bundle, has a very limited effect, if any, on the stability of the knee, and is almost undetectable clinically.
(2) A complete tear of the ACL has a significant effect on the anterior translation of the tibia, as detectable by the Lachman test, and a limited effect on the internal rotation of the tibia in both static and dynamic (pivot shift) conditions.
(3) The ALL has a very important role in controlling tibial internal rotation.
(4) Tears of the ALL always increase the severity of rotational instability and are the most important factor in eliciting an explosive pivot shift test result.

During the first 10 years of this century, mainly thanks to the studies of the University of Pittsburgh and Freddie Fu et al. [20], the double bundle ACL reconstruction technique was introduced. This technique was based on previous biomechanical studies, which had already shown that the anteromedial (AM) bundle controlled anterior tibial translation, while the posterolateral (PL) controlled internal rotation and the pivot shift [21].

To verify the efficacy of the double bundle technique, we performed an in vivo biomechanical study with the use of a navigation system, where we compared the double bundle technique with anatomic single bundle ACL reconstruction combined with an extra-articular procedure. This study was published in Knee Surgery Sports Traumatology and Arthroscopy and prestigiously commented on by Ejnar Eriksson in the commentary entitled "Double bundle or single bundle plus extra-articular tenodesis in ACL reconstruction?"[22]

In this study, we demonstrated that:

(1) The addition of a second bundle (PL) to an anatomic single bundle (AM) does not significantly affect the internal rotation of the tibia.
(2) The addition of lateral extra-articular reconstruction to standard anatomic single bundle ACL reconstruction is more effective than the double bundle technique in controlling internal tibial rotation and the pivot shift (Tables 3.6 and 3.7).

Table 3.6 Double bundle reconstruction: the mean AP tibial displacement (mm), internal rotation (°), and external rotation (°) before ACL reconstruction, after anatomic AM bundle fixation and after PL bundle fixation (AM+PL). Red Square: $p < 0.05$

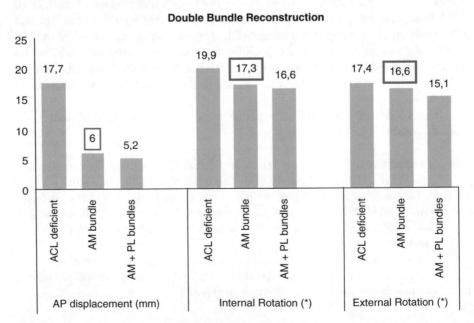

Table 3.7 Single bundle reconstruction and lateral tenodesis: the mean AP tibial displacement (mm), the internal rotation (°), and the external rotation (°) before ACL reconstruction, after single bundle (SB) reconstruction and after SB reconstruction and lateral tenodesis. Red Square: $p < 0.05$

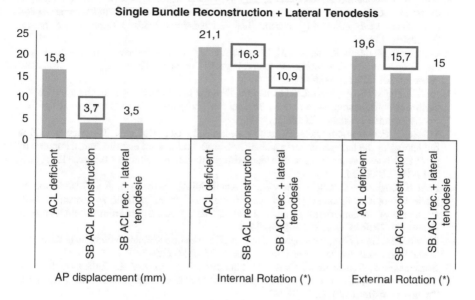

We can postulate that the success of the double bundle reconstruction, as proposed by Freddie Fu, is limited to the cases where the first bundle is vertically, and not anatomically, positioned.

In fact, most of the following studies never reported any clinical advantages of double bundle reconstruction compared to anatomical single bundle reconstruction [23, 24].

References

1. Tanaka M, Vyas D, Moloney G, Bedi A, Pearle AD, Musahl V. What does it take to have a high-grade pivot shift? Knee Surg Sports Traumatol Arthrosc. 2012;20(4):737–42.
2. Hughston JC, Andrews JR, Cross MJ, Moschi A. Classification of knee ligament instabilities. Part II. The lateral compartment. J Bone Joint Surg Am. 1976;58(2):173–9.
3. Schindler OS. Surgery for anterior cruciate ligament deficiency: a historical perspective. Knee Surg Sports Traumatol Arthrosc. 2012;20(1):5–47.
4. Edwards D, Villar R. Anterior cruciate ligament injury. Practitioner. 1993;237(1523):113–4.116–7
5. Monaco E, Ferretti A, Labianca L, Maestri B, Speranza A, Kelly MJ, et al. Navigated knee kinematics after cutting of the ACL and its secondary restraint. Knee Surg Sports Traumatol Arthrosc. 2012;20(5):870–7.
6. Claes S, Vereecke E, Maes M, Victor J, Verdonk P, Bellemans J. Anatomy of the anterolateral ligament of the knee. J Anat. 2013;223(4):321–8.
7. Claes S, Neven E, Callewaert B, Desloovere K, Bellemans J. Tibial rotation in single- and double-bundle ACL reconstruction: a kinematic 3-D in vivo analysis. Knee Surg Sports Traumatol Arthrosc. 2011;19(Suppl 1):S115–21.

8. Pearle AD, Solomon DJ, Wanich T, Moreau-Gaudry A, Granchi CC, Wickiewicz TL, et al. Reliability of navigated knee stability examination: a cadaveric evaluation. Am J Sports Med. 2007;35(8):1315–20.
9. Woo SL-Y, Kanamori A, Zeminski J, Yagi M, Papageorgiou C, Fu FH. The effectiveness of reconstruction of the anterior cruciate ligament with hamstrings and patellar tendon. A cadaveric study comparing anterior tibial and rotational loads. J Bone Joint Surg Am. 2002;84(6):907–14.
10. Caterine S, Litchfield R, Johnson M, Chronik B, Getgood A. A cadaveric study of the antero-lateral ligament: re-introducing the lateral capsular ligament. Knee Surg Sports Traumatol Arthrosc. 2015;23(11):3186–95.
11. Iorio R, Pagnottelli M, Vadalà A, Giannetti S, Di Sette P, Papandrea P, et al. Open-wedge high tibial osteotomy: comparison between manual and computer-assisted techniques. Knee Surg Sports Traumatol Arthrosc. 2013;21(1):113–9.
12. Monaco E, Fabbri M, Mazza D, Daggett M, Redler A, Lanzetti RM, et al. The effect of sequential tearing of the anterior cruciate and anterolateral ligament on anterior translation and the pivot-shift phenomenon: A cadaveric study using navigation. Arthrosc J Arthrosc Relat Surg. 2018;34(4):1009–14.
13. Ferretti A, Monaco E, Gaj E, Andreozzi V, Annibaldi A, Carrozzo A, et al. Risk factors for grade 3 pivot shift in knees with acute anterior cruciate ligament injuries: A comprehensive evaluation of the importance of osseous and soft tissue parameters from the SANTI Study Group. Am J Sports Med. 2020;48(10):2408–17.
14. Parsons EM, Gee AO, Spiekerman C, Cavanagh PR. The biomechanical function of the antero-lateral ligament of the knee. Am J Sports Med. 2015;43(3):669–74.
15. Bonanzinga T, Signorelli C, Grassi A, Lopomo N, Bragonzoni L, Zaffagnini S, et al. Kinematics of ACL and anterolateral ligament. Part I: Combined lesion. Knee Surg Sports Traumatol Arthrosc. 2017;25(4):1055–61.
16. Spencer L, Burkhart TA, Tran MN, Rezansoff AJ, Deo S, Caterine S, et al. Biomechanical analysis of simulated clinical testing and reconstruction of the anterolateral ligament of the knee. Am J Sports Med. 2015;43(9):2189–97.
17. Johnson LL. Lateral capsualr ligament complex: anatomical and surgical considerations. Am J Sports Med. giugno. 1979;7(3):156–60.
18. Wroble RR, Grood ES, Cummings JS, Henderson JM, Noyes FR. The role of the lateral extraarticular restraints in the anterior cruciate ligament-deficient knee. Am J Sports Med. 1993;21(2):257–62. discussion 263
19. Kittl C, El-Daou H, Athwal KK, Gupte CM, Weiler A, Williams A, et al. The role of the antero-lateral structures and the ACL in controlling laxity of the intact and ACL-deficient knee. Am J Sports Med. 2016;44(2):345–54.
20. Yagi M, Wong EK, Kanamori A, Debski RE, Fu FH, Woo SL-Y. Biomechanical analysis of an anatomic anterior cruciate ligament reconstruction. Am J Sports Med. 2002;30(5):660–6.
21. Furman W, Marshall JL, Girgis FG. The anterior cruciate ligament. A functional analysis based on postmortem studies. J Bone Joint Surg Am. 1976;58(2):179–85.
22. Monaco E, Labianca L, Conteduca F, De Carli A, Ferretti A. Double bundle or single bundle plus extraarticular tenodesis in ACL reconstruction? A CAOS study. Knee Surg Sports Traumatol Arthrosc. 2007;15(10):1168–74.
23. Oh J-Y, Kim K-T, Park Y-J, Won H-C, Yoo J-I, Moon D-K, et al. Biomechanical comparison of single-bundle versus double-bundle anterior cruciate ligament reconstruction: a meta-analysis. Knee Surg Relat Res. 2020;32(1):14.
24. Torkaman A, Yazdi H, Hosseini MG. The results of single bundle versus double bundle ACL reconstruction surgery, a retrospective study and review of literature. Med Arch Sarajevo Bosnia Herzeg. 2016;70(5):351–3.

Surgical Anatomy in ACL Tears

4

Andrea Ferretti and Andrea Redler

In the previous chapters, we carefully described the anatomy and biomechanics of the anterolateral complex of the knee, particularly focusing on the anatomy and the role of the anterolateral ligament in the pathogenesis of anterolateral rotatory instability (ALRI) and the pivot shift phenomenon.

Another crucial aspect worthy of being thoroughly investigated and analysed in this chapter is the real involvement of the anterolateral complex in ACL tears and how often its injuries occur in current clinical practice.

To carefully investigate this issue, when studying the actual involvement of the anterolateral complex in the framework of ACL injuries, the most reliable sample is represented by acute injuries. At this stage, not only are the injuries easily detectable during surgery, but they are also likely linked to the initial trauma; all other tears or injuries that possibly occurred as a result of new giving-way episodes, joint instability, progressive stretching or any functional overload associated with ACL insufficiency can be reasonably excluded.

In the past, at the beginning of the modern era of knee surgery and until the late eighties, when knee surgery was still carried out through open techniques without the aid of an arthroscope and femoral tunnelling was inevitably made through an outside-in technique, exploring the external compartment was a standard practice [1]. Furthermore, according to the rules at that time, surgery at the acute stage of the injury was recommended on a large scale, as the repair and reconstruction of peripheral structures and of the ACL itself was technically easier only when an early operation was performed within a few days or weeks of the initial injury.

Moreover, early surgery was strongly encouraged, as it would result in a higher rate of repairable meniscal tears and a lower prevalence of cartilage and meniscal

A. Ferretti (✉) · A. Redler
Orthopaedic Unit, Sant'Andrea University Hospital, La Sapienza University, Rome, Italy

© The Author(s), under exclusive license to Springer Nature Switzerland AG 2022
A. Ferretti (ed.), *Anterolateral Rotatory Instability in ACL Deficient Knee*, https://doi.org/10.1007/978-3-031-00115-4_4

tears, resulting in a lower risk of late degenerative osteoarthrosis (DOA) [2]. With the rise of arthroscopy and the spread of arthroscopic-assisted ACL reconstructions with minimally invasive techniques, surgeons have progressively focused increasingly on the ACL. Other structures, including the anterolateral capsule and ligaments, that were not visible with an arthroscope soon became neglected and disappeared from a comprehensive description of the surgical anatomy of ACL tears. As a result, the most popular technique soon became single-incision arthroscopy-assisted ACL reconstruction with the patellar tendon, performed through inside-out femoral tunnelling in a nonanatomical vertical position (Rosenberg's technique) [3]. It took decades to realize how irrational the method was, based on inappropriate use of an incredibly useful tool, i.e. the arthroscope; in actual fact arthroscopy itself, like other revolutionary discoveries, caused some collateral damage. Moreover, due to the high risk of postoperative stiffness and arthrofibrosis observed as a result of BPTB ACL reconstruction performed soon after injury (acute phase), most surgeons suggested that a delayed operation be performed once the early posttraumatic inflammatory phase was resolved, and a full range of motion was regained [4]. As a result, acute ACL reconstruction became very unusual, and an entire generation of young surgeons lost any chances to comprehensively understand the actual surgical anatomy of ACL tears.

In contrast, since we moved to the new hospital, the entire emergency department was organized to recognize and treat all acute ACL tears requiring surgery early. Thanks to our original approach to acute ACL injuries, a prospective study on the surgical findings of ACL tears was started, allowing us to develop one of the largest worldwide experiences of ACL reconstructions performed within two weeks of the first injury. Furthermore, as our preferred technique still included a second incision on the lateral side for either outside-in femoral drilling or the inspection of the anterolateral compartment, the anterolateral complex was actually inspected in most cases.

Our first study on the surgical anatomy of ACL tears dates back to 2017, when, after a long pathway of submissions, reviews, resubmissions and a final rejection by the KSSTA, followed by lively controversy with the editor, other members of the editorial board, and reviewers, it was finally published in "Arthroscopy". In this paper [5], we presented our first consecutive series of acute ACL injuries with regular exploration of the anterolateral complex and an accurate description of the surgical anatomy. Nonetheless, at the end of the year, our study was the most quoted study in this prestigious scientific journal.

In a series of sixty cases of ACL injuries, which supposedly appeared to be isolated, with positive Lachman and Pivot Shift tests carried out under anaesthesia in the operating room, exploration of the external compartment made it possible to detect the presence of a macroscopically visible injury in the anterolateral capsular complex just beneath the fascia lata in 54 cases (90%). The fascia lata itself appeared as normal, just slightly stretched or mildly haemorrhagic but perfectly inserted to the Gerdy's tubercle in all cases (Fig. 4.1).

The patterns of ALL and capsular injuries were also classified into the following 4 types [5] (Fig. 4.2):

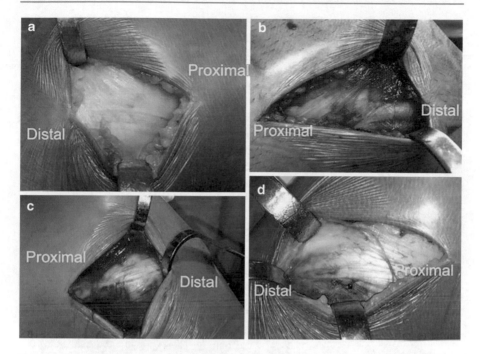

Fig. 4.1 The fascia lata as it can appear in anterolateral complex injuries: (**a**) Normal; (**b, c**) Mildly stretched and haemorrhagic; (**d**) Moderately stretched and haemorrhagic. In all cases, the iliotibial tract is normally attached to Gerdy's tubercle

- Type I (19 cases, 31.7%): injury characterized by visible lengthening with haemorrhagic infiltration located on the distal and anterior portions of the ALL (incomplete injury) (Fig. 4.3a1–3)
- Type II (16 cases, 26.7%): injury comparable to type 1 but more extended. The injury included the anterolateral capsule, the proximal portion of the ligament and the posterolateral capsule (incomplete injury) (Fig. 4.3b1–3)
- Type III (13 cases, 21.6%): complete ALL injury, generally located on the distal portion of the ALL, below the lateral meniscus and just above the tibial plateau (Fig. 4.3c1–3)
- Type IV (6 cases, 10%) injury characterized by insertional detachment (avulsion) with a bone fragment at the level of the margin of lateral tibial plateau (Segond's fracture)

To find comparable data, we had to refer to studies in the seventies when similar findings were reported by several authors. Hughston et al. [6], in a series of six cases of acute ALRI, reported injury of the middle third of the lateral capsular ligament in five cases. Mueller [7], in addition to recognizing the role of the anterolateral femoral ligament as the first structure involved in ALRI, described how its injuries were mostly confined to the posterior inner aspect, being either a visible avulsion from the femur or the overstretching of its femorotibial fibres. Similarly, Terry et al. [8], in a series of eighty-two cases of knee ligament injuries classified as anteromedial-anterolateral rotatory instability, reported that injuries of deep and superficial layers of the iliotibial tract occurred in 93% of the cases. Later, Puddu [9] stated that in ALRI, injuries to the anterolateral capsule occur in all cases, along with ACL tears.

After many decades, our abovementioned study brought surgeons' attention back to a long-hidden aspect (ever since the introduction of arthroscopy). Although the results were not essentially different from those reported in the seventies and eighties, this study aroused interest in the scientific community, as it reaffirmed the fact that an isolated ACL injury is an extremely rare event.

In the following years, the collection of data concerning surgical findings in acute ACL injuries has been ongoing, and recently, the results of a consecutive series of 200 cases were reported [10]. This probably represents the most conspicuous case history ever published on this kind of injury. In this study, all injuries associated with ACL tears were reported. Moreover, even the bone structure

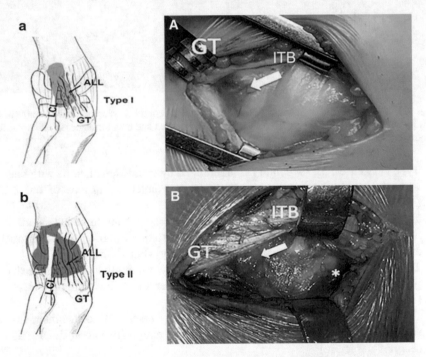

Fig. 4.2 Pattern of injuries of the anterolateral capsule in acute ACL tears. (**a**) Type I lesion: multilevel rupture in which individual layers are torn at different levels with macroscopic haemorrhage involving the area of the anterolateral ligament (ALL) and extended to the anterolateral capsule only (white arrow). (**b**) Type II lesion: multilevel rupture in which individual layers are torn at different levels with macroscopic haemorrhage extended from the area of the ALL and capsule (white arrow) to the posterolateral capsule (*). (**c**) Type III lesion: complete transverse tear involving the area of the ALL near its insertion to the lateral tibial plateau, always distal to the lateral meniscus. (**d**) Type IV lesion: bony avulsion (Segond's fracture). (Drawings courtesy of Angelo de Carli). *ALL* anterolateral ligament, *GT* Gerdy's tubercle, *LCL* lateral collateral ligament, *SF* Segond's fracture

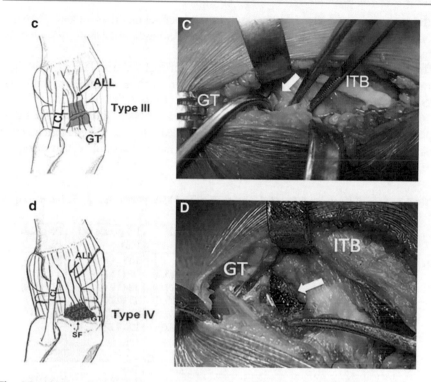

Fig. 4.2 (continued)

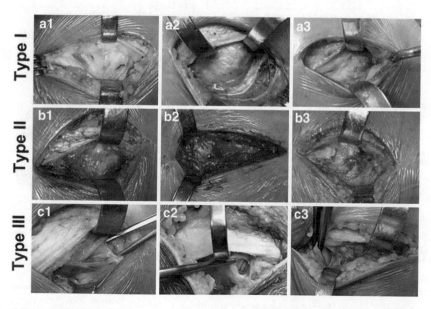

Fig. 4.3 (**a, b, c**) The different types of lesions are described. Segond's fracture (Type IV) will be better described in the next chapter. (**a2, a3, b3, c1, c2** Right Knee. **a1, b1, b2, c3** Left Knee)

of the joint was analysed to investigate its possible effect on the pivot shift phenomenon; the tibial slope, meniscal slope, and femoral condylar morphology were evaluated with MRI.

In addition to confirming the high prevalence of ALL injuries (90%) with eight percent of Segond's fractures, in this study a high prevalence of injuries of either the lateral and medial meniscus or both were reported (Table 4.1).

As a result of a particularly accurate statistical analysis, the most interesting aspect of this study was that, among all the variables (associated ligamentous injuries, meniscal injuries, skeletal structure), the only factor that could cause an explosive pivot shift was the presence of an ALL injury.

Table 4.1 Rate of identified associated injuries, stratified by explosive (grade 3) and nonexplosive (grades 1–2) pivot shift

		Total (%)	PS grade 1-2 (%)	PS grade 3 (%)
AL lesion	n	200	165	35
	No lesion	26 (13.0)	26 (15.8)	2 (5.7)
	Incomplete tear of the AL capsule	34 (17.0)	32 (19.4)	21 (60.0)
	Incomplete tear of the AL and PL capsule	66 (33.0)	45 (27.3)	8 (22.9)
	Complete tear	58 (29.0)	50 (30.3)	4 (11.4)
	Segond's fracture	16 (8.0)	12 (7.3)	
AL lesion (Y/N)	n	200	165	35
	Yes	174	139 (84.2)	35 (100)
	No	(87.0)	26 (15.8)	
		26 (13.0)		
MCL	n	200	165	35
	0 mm	174	146 (88.5)	28 (80.0)
	0–5 mm	(87.0)	11 (6.7)	5 (14.3)
	5–10 mm	16 (8.0)	6 (3.6)	1 (2.9)
	>10 mm	7 (3.5)	2 (1.2)	1 (2.9)
		3 (1.5)		
MCL (Y/N)	n	200	165	35
	Yes	26 (13.0)	19 (11.5)	7 (20.0)
	No	174	146 (88.5)	28 (80.0)
		(87.0)		
Outerbridge	n	200	165	35
	0	191	157 (95.2)	34 (97.1)
	Grade 1 MFC	(95.5)	6 (3.6)	1(2.9)
	Grade 2 MFC	7 (3.5)	1 (0.6)	
	Grade 2 LFC	1 (0.5)	1 (0.6)	
		1 (0.5)		
Outer bridge (Y/N)	n	200	165	35
	Yes	9 (4.5)	8 (4.8)	1 (2.9)
	No	191	157 (95.2)	34 (97.1)
		(95.5)		

Table 4.1 (continued)

		Total (%)	PS grade 1–2 (%)	PS grade 3 (%)
Medial meniscal tears				
	n	200	165	35
	No Lesion	147	119 (72.1)	28 (80.0)
	Bucket handle	(73.5)	3 (1.8)	1 (2.9)
	Longitudinal anterior	3 (1.5)	4 (2.4)	5 (14.3)
	horn	5 (2.5)	16 (9.7)	1 (2.9)
	Longitudinal	21	4 (2.4)	
	posterior horn	(10.5)	19 (11.5)	
	Radial body lesion	5 (2.5)		
	Ramp lesion	19 (9.5)		
Medial meniscal tears (y/n)	n	200	165	35
	Yes	53	46 (27.9)	7 (20.0)
	No	(26.5)	119 (72.1)	28 (80.0)
		147		
		(73.5)		
Lateral meniscal tears	n	200	165	35
	No Lesion	140	115 (69.7)	25 (71.4)
	Flap handle	(70.0)	2 (1.2)	1 (2.9)
	Longitudinal anterior	3 (1.5)	12 (7.3)	3 (8.6)
	horn	15 (7.5)	2 (1.2)	2 (5.7)
	Longitudinal	4 (2.0)	21(12.7)	3 (8.6)
	posterior horn	24	13(7.9)	1 (2.9)
	Radial body lesion	(12.0)		
	Root lesion	14 (7.0)		
Lateral meniscal tears (y/n)	n	200	165	35
	Yes	60	50 (30.3)	10 (28.6)
	No	(30.0)	115 (69.7)	25 (71.4)
		140		
		(70.0)		
Medial and lateral meniscal tears (y/n)	n	200	165	35
	Yes	5 (2.5)	5 (3.0)	35 (100.0)
	No	195	160 (97.0)	
		(97.5)		

AL anterolateral, *MCL* medial collateral ligament, *MFC* medial femoral condyle, *LFC* lateral femoral condyle, *PL* posterolateral, *PS* pivot shift

This aspect has also been confirmed by a previous study [11], in which a significant reduction in the pivot shift can be achieved, in acute cases, as a result of ALL repair only, despite a concomitant ACL tear.

This long-lasting effort of data analysis and collection regarding a unique case series firmly confirmed the crucial role of secondary restraint injuries in the pathogenesis of anterolateral rotatory laxity and the pivot shift phenomenon.

References

1. Norwood LA Jr, Andrews JR, Meisterling RC, Glancy GL. Acute anterolateral rotatory instability of the knee. J Bone Joint Surg Am. 1979;61(5):704–9.
2. Prodromidis AD, Drosatou C, Thivaios GC, Zreik N, Charalambous CP. Timing of anterior cruciate ligament reconstruction and relationship with meniscal tears: a systematic review and meta-analysis. Am J Sports Med. 2020;9:363546520964486. https://doi.org/10.1177/0363546520964486. Epub ahead of print. PMID: 33166481
3. Rosenberg TD, Brown GC, Deffner KT. Anterior cruciate ligament reconstruction with a quadrupled semi- tendinosus autograft. Sports Med Arthrosc Rev. 1997;5:51–8.
4. Akgün I, Ogüt T, Kesmezacar H, Yücel I. Central third bone-patellar tendon-bone arthroscopic anterior cruciate ligament reconstruction: a 4-year follow-up. J Knee Surg. 2002;15(4):207–12.
5. Ferretti A, Monaco E, Fabbri M, Maestri B, De Carli A. Prevalence and classification of injuries of anterolateral complex in acute anterior cruciate ligament tears. Arthrosc J Arthrosc Relat Surg. 2016:1–8. https://doi.org/10.1016/j.arthro.2016.05.010.
6. Hughston JC, Andrews JR, Cross MJ, Moschi A. Classification of knee ligament instabilities. Part I. The medial compartment and cruciate ligaments. J Bone Joint Surg Am. 1976;58(2):159–72.
7. Muller W. The Knee. New York: Springer Verlang.
8. Terry GC, Norwood LA, Hughston JC, Caldwell KM. How iliotibial tract injuries of the knee combine with acute anterior cruciate ligament tears to influence abnormal anterior tibial displacement. Am J Sports Med. 1993;21(1):55–60.
9. Puddu G, Ferretti A, Mariani PP, Conteduca F. Le lesioni isolate del legamento crociato anteriore. Il Ginocchio. 1987;VI. Atti del VII Corso
10. Ferretti A, Gaj E, Andreozzi V, Sonnery-cottet B, Saithna A. Risk factors for grade 3 pivot shift in knees with acute anterior cruciate ligament injuries: a comprehensive evaluation of the importance of osseous and soft tissue parameters from the SANTI study group. Am J Sports Med. 2020;48(10):2408–17.
11. Monaco E, Ferretti A, Labianca L, Maestri B, Speranza A, Kelly MJ, D'Arrigo C. Navigated knee kinematics after cutting of the ACL and its secondary restraint. Knee Surg Sports Traumatol Arthrosc. 2012;20(5):870–7.

The Segond's Fracture

5

Andrea Ferretti, Edoardo Gaj, and Daniele Mazza

Avulsion fracture involving the proximal tibia just distal to the lateral plateau was first described in 1879 by a French surgeon, Paul Segond, after performing cadaveric experiments [1]. The author described a resistant, pearly, fibrous band in the lateral compartment of the knee, whose traction resulted in a cortical avulsion of the lateral proximal tibia. This injury was named Segond's fracture, and several studies have demonstrated an association of this fracture with anterior cruciate ligament (ACL) tears, meniscal tears, damage to structures of the posterolateral corner and other avulsion injuries [2]. Currently, it might seem strange, almost bizarre, how Segond's fracture, which was described well before the discovery of X-rays by Wilhelm Roentgen in 1896, has become popular as an indirect radiological sign of an ACL injury over time (Fig. 5.1). Today, although Segond's fracture can be associated with other knee injuries, if it is present, the ACL should be considered torn until proven otherwise.

The precise pathogenesis of Segond's fracture has been the subject of debate, partially due to the complexity of the anterolateral capsuloligamentous anatomy. Paul Segond demonstrated that internal rotation and varus stress applied to the knee causes tension on the lateral joint capsule at its midpoint; he believed that a resistant band of tissue produces an avulsion fracture of the lateral tibial plateau posterior to the insertion of the iliotibial tract on Gerdy's tubercle.

In a recent descriptive study [3] on the pattern and prevalence of injuries of the lateral capsule occurring along with acute ACL tears, Ferretti et al. found that among the overall 90% prevalence of injuries involving the anterolateral complex, Segond's fracture occurs in approximately 10% of cases. In a more extended experience related to more than 200 cases of acute ACL tears, the true prevalence of Segond's fractures decreased to approximately 8% [4]. Based on these findings, it was postulated that this avulsion fracture represents the tip of the iceberg of anterolateral

A. Ferretti (✉) · E. Gaj · D. Mazza
Orthopaedic Unit, Sant'Andrea University Hospital, La Sapienza University, Rome, Italy

© The Author(s), under exclusive license to Springer Nature Switzerland AG 2022
A. Ferretti (ed.), *Anterolateral Rotatory Instability in ACL Deficient Knee*,
https://doi.org/10.1007/978-3-031-00115-4_5

Fig. 5.1 Segond's fracture
on X-rays

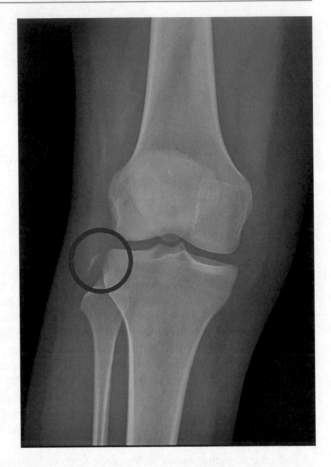

capsule and ligament lesions, occurring along with ACL tears and possibly affecting
the rotational stability of the knee.

Moreover, Claes et al. [5], as a result of their study on the anterolateral ligament
(ALL), whose insertion lies on the proximal tibia, where Segond's fracture consis-
tently avulses, suggested that Segond's fracture is actually a bony avulsion of the
ALL. A similar finding was provided by John Feagin in his textbook "The Crucial
Ligaments" (see Chap. 2, Fig. 2.3) [6].

5.1 Biomechanics

Many anatomical and biomechanical studies have focused on the anterolateral capsule and ALL [7–10]. Meanwhile, their roles as the secondary restraints of the ACL
in controlling tibial internal rotation and the pivot shift phenomenon are still
debated. Surprisingly, all previous studies that focused on the anatomy and function
of soft tissues, including ligaments and capsules, whose dissection was performed
by various authors, have reported conflicting results [11–13]. In 2017, we published

the first and, to our knowledge, the only biomechanical study on the effect of an experimentally reproduced Segond's fracture on knee stability in an ACL-deficient knee [14].

The biomechanical cadaver study was conducted on entire fresh frozen cadavers following the same protocol used for evaluating the effect of sequential tearing of the ACL and ALL on anteroposterior (AP) translation, combined external and internal rotation (axial tibial rotation), the Lachman test and pivot shift test, with the aid of navigation [15]. The navigation system was equipped with dedicated software that could perform accurate static and real-time dynamic measurements by means of wires strongly fixed to the bone. All tests and navigation processes were performed by the same experienced surgeon. Three different conditions were tested: an intact knee, an ACL-deficient knee and a knee with an ACL injury with Segond's fracture (Fig. 5.2).

Static measurements of anterior tibial translation (ATT) and axial tibial rotation (ATR) at 30° of flexion were performed in all three conditions. All measurements were recorded under a manual maximum force applied by the same surgeon who made every effort to apply a similar load to the knee to minimize intra-observer variability.

Dynamic measurements of ATT and ATR during the pivot shift test were also performed under the same three conditions. ATT was expressed in millimetres and ATR was expressed in degrees, and a diagram showing the curve of ATT and ATR during the test was visualized and saved as a screenshot at the end of each procedure step. All data were collected and statistically analysed by a single researcher.

As shown in Tables 5.1, 5.2, 5.3 and 5.4, an isolated complete tear of the ACL had a significant effect only on ATT and only a mild effect, if any, on the rotational stability of the knee; the addition of a reproduced Segond's fracture had a significant effect on ATR in both static and dynamic conditions during the execution of the pivot shift test. Therefore, from a biomechanical point of view, a Segond's fracture has the same effect as a severe injury on the ALL, both of which usually occur along with an ACL tear.

Fig. 5.2 Segond's fracture as reproduced on a cadaver model

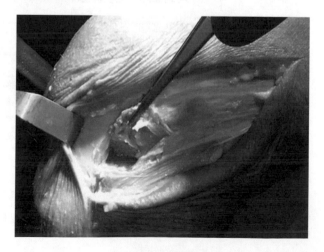

Table 5.1 Anterior tibial translation during pivot shift (Dynamic measurements)

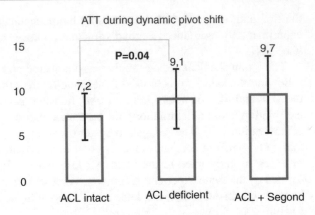

Table 5.2 Axial tibial rotation (Internal+External tibial rotation) during pivot shift (Dynamic measurements)

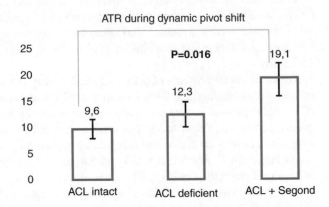

Table 5.3 Anterior tibial translation (ATT) during pivot shift (Static measurements)

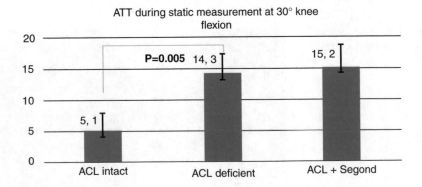

Table 5.4 Axial tibial rotation (Internal+External tibial rotation) (Static measurements)

ATR during statisc measurement at 30° knee flexion

	P=0.005	
		30,9
	26,9	
20,7		
ACL intact	ACL deficient	ACL + Segond

Recently, Mullins et al. performed a cadaver study [16] investigating the bone density of various entheses of the proximal tibia using a micro-CT scan to perform "virtual biopsies", to measure the bone trabecular volume fraction ("bone volume divided by the total volume" (BV/TV)). The subentheseal trabecular properties at Segond's site were compared with other entheses across the tibial plateau and fibular head, and it was hypothesized that a lower trabecular bone structure at Segond's site would explain its propensity for avulsion. A reduced mineral content (BV/TV), which correlates with tensile and torsional strength, was detected in the anterolateral aspect of the tibia exactly where Segond's fracture usually occurs, possibly resulting in a weaker bone. Based on their results, the authors postulated that the high prevalence of Segond's fracture was due to a reduced mineral content, actually questioning the existence of the ALL, postulating that according to Frost's Mechanostat hypothesis, the insertion of a ligament would correspond to a stronger and more resistant site.

However, to better understand the mechanism and biomechanics of a Segond's fracture, additional factors should be reasonably considered.

In fact, in their study, the authors compared virtual biopsies of several entheses of various ligaments and tendons with different biomechanical properties. Therefore, it was not surprising that the entheses themselves showed different properties. In particular, the ultimate failure load and the stiffness of the ALL were much lower than those of all other ligaments and tendons whose bony insertion was evaluated [17–19]. Compared with the ACL, Lateral Collateral Ligament (LCL) and iliotibial band (ITB), the biomechanical properties of the ALL are more than ten times lower [20, 21], not to mention the difference with the patellar tendon [22]. Therefore, we should not be surprised if a similar difference was found in their sites of insertion. Moreover, the ALL is only a secondary restraint of internal rotation, with the ACL being the first restraint [23]. Therefore, the ALL usually exerts tension over its insertion only as the result of an ACL tear. Compared with other, stronger entheses, ALL insertion is probably not normally exerted, with a resulting lack of the constant and adequate stimulus required for an adaptive bony reaction and hypertrophy.

In conclusion, while the study of Mullins et al. reasonably explained how a Segond's fracture, even if a rare event, is probably the most frequent avulsion fracture of the tibial plateau, it does not challenge the hypothesis of the existence of a discrete ligament (the ALL) that is strong enough to sometimes pull out its bony insertion as a result of forced internal rotation and ACL failure.

5.2   Surgical Anatomy

As Segond's fracture occurs in less than 10% of acute ACL tear, cases collecting a reliable series of cases would mean having access to hundreds of cases of truly acute ACL tears. In fact, the literature is scarce, and most of the papers are case reports or observational studies of a few randomly collected cases [24].

Between 2014 and 2020, in a consecutive series of 210 acute patients prospectively selected and admitted for early surgical treatment, 17 were diagnosed as having a Segond's fracture. In addition to X-rays, MRI and/or CT scans confirmed the anterolateral location of the bony avulsion (Figs. 5.1, 5.2, and 5.3).

Although the size of bony fragments is usually small, a few cases of exceptionally large fragments have been reported as a result of severe knee injuries of polytrauma (Figs. 5.3 and 5.4).

During preoperative evaluation under anaesthesia, the Lachman test and pivot shift test were always positive, confirming the anterolateral pattern of the instability. In contrast, the varus test at either 30° of flexion or in extension was negative in all cases.

Preliminary diagnostic arthroscopy showed a complete rupture of the ACL in all cases. Along with standard ACL reconstruction with the hamstrings, the lateral compartment was explored to detect the fracture, which was surgically inspected, accurately described, and photographically documented. With the knee flexed on the operating table, the lateral compartment was approached through a hockey stick skin incision. Below the subcutaneous tissue, the fascia lata was exposed and carefully examined: it was slightly haemorrhagic in 9 cases, only haemorrhagic in 5 cases, and haemorrhagic, attenuated and stretched in 3 cases (Fig. 5.5).

It was normally inserted on Gerdy's tibial tubercle in all cases. The deeper, capsular layer was exposed by splitting the fascia lata along its fibres: the capsule was found to be diffusely haemorrhagic and frankly stretched in all cases; the bony fragment was always detected at the proximal tibia just below the lateral meniscus, almost midway between Gerdy's tubercle and the anterior edge of the fibular head.

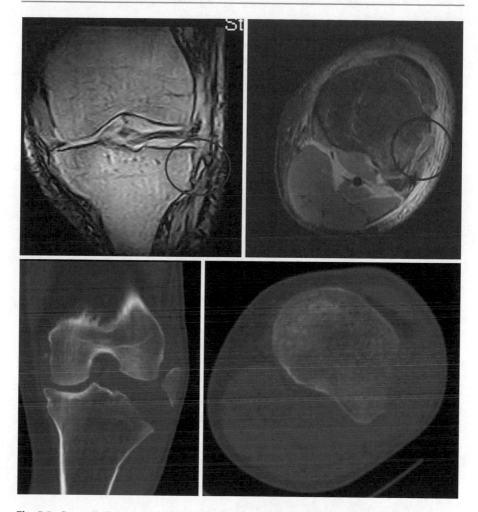

Fig. 5.3 Segond's fracture on MRI and CT in axial and coronal view

The size of the fragment was variable but always corresponded to the preoperative imaging; the ALL and the surrounding capsule were the only structures attached to the bony fragment in all cases (Fig. 5.6). In fact, the site of the fragment corresponded to the site of insertion of the ALL, as described by Claes et al. [5].

Based on our surgical findings of the largest ever-reported case series of Segond's fractures, we can reasonably state that Segond's fractures:

(1) are constantly associated with a complete rupture of the ACL resulting in anterolateral rotatory instability (ALRI)
(2) represent the avulsion of the tibial insertion of the ALL

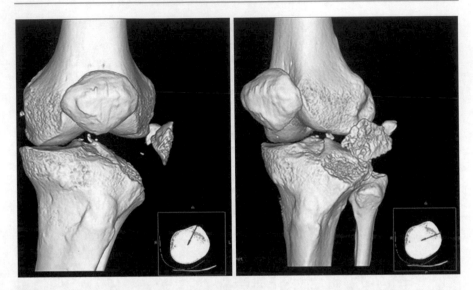

Fig. 5.4 Exceptionally large and rare Segond's fracture on CT and 3D CT

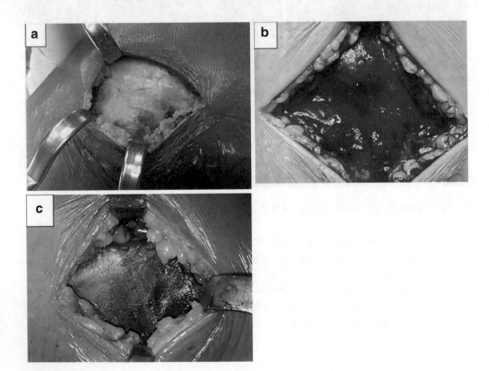

Fig. 5.5 Fascia lata as it can appear in case of Segond's fracture: (**a**) *Mildly haemorrhagic;* (**b**) *Haemorrhagic;* (**c**) *Haemorrhagic and stretched*

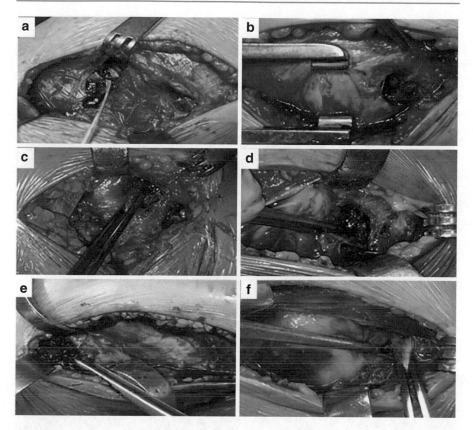

Fig. 5.6 In our series, the Segond's fracture was always identified at the tibial insertion of ALL. Detachment of fascia lata, biceps tendon or other lateral structures was never encountered. (**a**, **e** Left Knee; **b**, **c**, **d**, **f** Right Knee)

However, it must be considered that in addition to the bony injury, the ALL itself and its whole anterolateral complex also underwent severe plastic deformation, as documented by the extensive haemorrhagic infarction associated with diffuse stretching, sometimes extending to the overlying ITB.

5.3 Surgical Treatment

Among the 17 cases of Segond's fracture that were observed and surgically treated in our hospital between 2014 and 2020, twelve were reviewed at a minimum follow-up of two years and were the subjects of recently published studies [25, 26]. Despite the relatively low number of patients, this series still represents the largest of this kind.

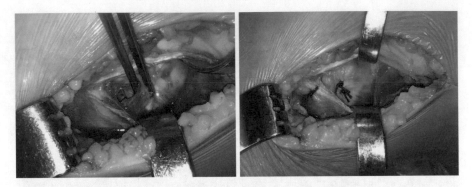

Fig. 5.7 Fixation of Segond's fracture using absorbable periosteal stitches

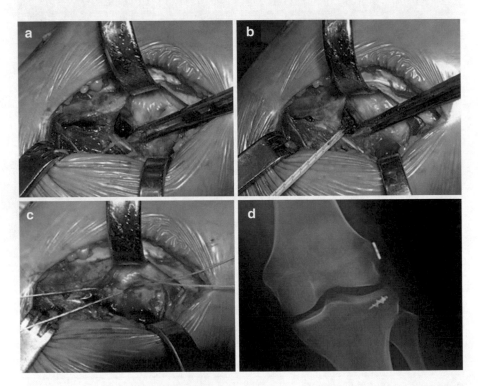

Fig. 5.8 Fixation of Segond's fracture using one suture anchor (**a**) identification of Segond's fracture (**b**) placement of the anchor suture (**c**) fixation of the bony fragment and re-tensioning of the antero-lateral capsule (**d**) post-operative x-ray after ACL reconstruction and Segond's fracture fixation

Once the bony fragment was identified, surgical repair consisted of the refixation of the fragment in its anatomical site by means of periosteal sutures in 11 cases, suture anchors in 5 cases and cancellous screws in one case where the bony fragment exceeded 2 cm in size. In all cases, the anterolateral complex was retensioned by plication using absorbable stitches (Figs. 5.7, 5.8, 5.9 and 5.10)

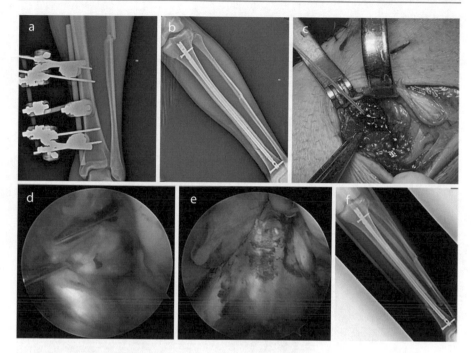

Fig. 5.9 A very unusual ski injury: open leg fracture associated with an ipsilateral ACL tear and Segond's fracture. Comprehensive one-stage treatment (fracture fixation, ACL and Segond's fracture repair). (**a**) *X-ray showing leg fracture after provisional external fixation;* (**b**) *X-ray after definitive intramedullary nailing before ACL and Segond's fracture repair;* (**c**) *Surgical finding after the first stage of the procedure (tibial fixation): Suture anchor repair of the Segond's fracture, identified as usual deep to the iliotibial tract and below the lateral meniscus;* (**d**) *Arthroscopy showing a repairable complete proximal ACL tear;* (**e**) *ACL tear as it appears after repair;* (**f**) *X-ray after comprehensive surgical treatment*

After repair and before intra-articular ACL reconstruction, the pivot shift test was repeated to verify the effect of the procedure. It was negative or only mildly positive (+—) in all cases. Therefore, the efficacy of the repair and the role of the Segond's fracture on anterolateral stability were confirmed.

As shown in Tables 5.5 and 5.6, which summarize the demographic data and preoperative and post-operative clinical findings, the results of the combined ACL reconstruction and Segond's fracture repair were excellent, with ten cases of IKDC with objective scores classified as A and two classified as B. No complications, such as infection, malunions, post-operative stiffness or arthrofibrosis, mechanical failure or rerupture of the ACL graft, were reported at a minimum follow-up of 2 years (mean: 28.6 ± 2.1 months). One patient underwent a second operation for meniscectomy. On average, the patients returned to the sport after six months. At the latest follow-up, all patients had returned to their preoperative sports activity level.

The main finding of this study was that repair of a Segond's fracture, performed along with standard ACL reconstruction with the hamstrings, is a safe and

Fig. 5.10 Fixation of Segond's fracture using a screw

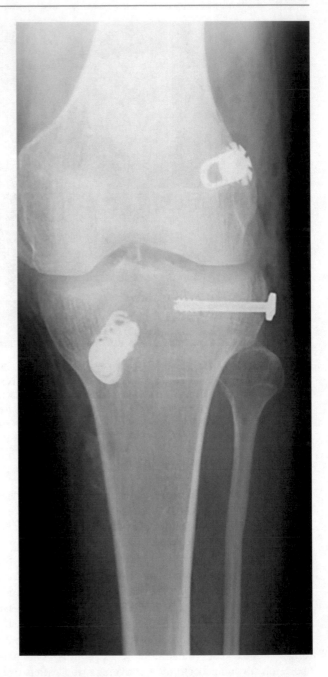

successful procedure resulting in the excellent recovery of knee stability and function and no major complications. Another important finding was that although a second skin incision and an open procedure are required, it does not otherwise increase morbidity. The patient post-operative course, rehabilitation and return to

Table 5.5 Demographic data

Male, n	10
Female, n	2
Affected knee, left, n	8
Affected knee, right, n	4
Weight, kg	58.3 ± 6.1 (range 48-71)
Age at procedure, y	26.5 ± 5.7 (range 16-45)
Interval to surgery (days)	4.5 ± 2.5 (range 2-7)
Follow-up period, m	28.6 ± 2.1 (range 24-37)
Additional procedures, n (%)	
Medial partial selective meniscectomy	4 (33%)
Lateral partial selective meniscectomy	1 (8%)
Lateral/medial selective meniscectomy	1 (8%)
Rerupture, n	0
Reintervention (meniscectomy), n	1

Table 5.6 Pre- and post-operative data

	Pre-operative	Post-operative	P
Joint Laxity (S-S), mm	10.2 ± 0.77 (range 9–11)	2.2 ± 0.7 (range 1–3)	<0.05
<3 mm	0	11 (92%)	
3–5 mm	4 (23%)	1 (8%)	
>5 mm	8 (67%)	0	
Lachman, n			<0.05
+	2	0	
++	3	0	
+++	7	0	
Pivot shift, n			<0.05
+	0	1 (8%)	
++	0	0	
+++	12 (100%)	0	
Lysholm	52.5 ± 5.1	91 ± 2.3	<0.05
Tegner	8.1 ± 1.1	7.1 ± 1.9	<0.05

the sport were identical to those occurring after isolated, standard intra-articular ACL reconstruction. Our results compare well with those of previous studies that reported that extra-articular reconstruction and/or repair, in addition to standard ACL reconstruction, has very good clinical outcomes and knee stability with a low rate of recurrence and failure [27–29].

Some authors have questioned the need to repair Segond's fractures, as their presence does not affect clinical results regardless of whether isolated ACL reconstruction is performed [30]. This finding is not surprising, as Segond's fractures do not necessarily increase the severity of anterolateral instability, possibly having the same effect as other unrecognized, misdiagnosed, and undetectable (by Xray) injuries of the ALL. If untreated, both bony and soft injuries could result in similar outcomes.

Our results confirm the importance of Segond's fractures and of the anterolateral ligament in controlling rotational stability of the knee and the pivot shift phenomenon, supporting early speculation that an unrecognized and/or untreated injury of an extra-articular structure such as the anterolateral complex may account for some cases of persistent rotational instability after isolated ACL reconstruction.

References

1. Segond P. Recherches cliniques et experimentales sur les epanchements sanguins du genou par entorse. Paris: Progres Medical; 1879.
2. Woods GW, Stanley RF, Tullos HS. Lateral capsular sign: x-ray clue to a significant knee instability. Am J Sports Med. 1979;7:27–33.
3. Ferretti A, Monaco E, Fabbri M, et al. Prevalence and classification of injuries of anterolateral complex in acute anterior cruciate ligament tears. Arthroscopy. 2017;33(1):147–54.
4. Ferretti A, Monaco E, Gaj E, et al. A. risk factors for grade 3 pivot shift in knees with acute anterior cruciate ligament injuries: a comprehensive evaluation of the importance of osseous and soft tissue parameters from the SANTI Study Group. Am J Sports Med. 2020;48(10):2408–17.
5. Claes S, Vereecke E, Maes M, et al. Anatomy of the anterolateral ligament of the knee. J Anat. 2013;223:321–8.
6. Feagin JA. The crucial ligaments. Churchill Livingstone; 1988.
7. Amis AA. Anterolateral knee biomechanics. Knee Surg Sports Traumatol Arthrosc. 2017;25(4):1015–23.
8. Corbo G, Norris M, Getgood A, et al. The infra-meniscal fibers of the anterolateral ligament are stronger and stiffer than the supra-meniscal fibers despite similar histological characteristics. Knee Surg Sports Traumatol Arthrosc. 2017;4:1078–85.
9. Getgood A, Brown C, Lording T, Amis A, Claes S, Geeslin A, Musahl V, ALC Consensus Group, et al. The anterolateral complex of the knee: results from the International ALC Consensus Group Meeting. Knee Surg Sports Traumatol Arthrosc. 2019;27(1):166–76.
10. Inderhaug E, Stephen JM, Williams A, et al. Biomechanical comparison of anterolateral procedures combined with anterior cruciate ligament reconstruction. Am J Sports Med. 2017;45(2):347–54.
11. Caterine S, Litchfield R, Johnson M, et al. A cadaveric study of the anterolateral ligament: re-introducing the lateral capsular ligament. Knee Surg Sports Traumatol Arthrosc. 2015;23(11):3186–95.
12. Redler A, Miglietta S, Monaco E, et al. Ultrastructural assessment of the anterolateral ligament. Orthop J Sports Med. 2019;7(12):2325967119887920.
13. Stijak L, Bumbaširević M, Radonjić V, et al. Anatomic description of the anterolateral ligament of the knee. Knee Surg Sports Traumatol Arthrosc. 2016;24(7):2083–8.
14. Monaco E, Mazza D, Redler A, et al. Segond's fracture: a biomechanical cadaveric study using navigation. J Orthop Traumatol. 2017;18(4):343–8.
15. Monaco E, Fabbri M, Mazza D, et al. The effect of sequential tearing of the anterior cruciate and anterolateral ligament on anterior translation and the pivot-shift phenomenon: a cadaveric study using navigation. Arthroscopy. 2018;34(4):1009–14.
16. Mullins W, Jarvis GE, Oluboyede D, et al. The Segond fracture occurs at the site of lowest subentheseal trabecular bone volume fraction on the tibial plateau. J Anat. 2020;237(6):1040–8.
17. Helito CP, Bonadio MB, Rozas JS, et al. Biomechanical study of strength and stiffness of the knee anterolateral ligament. BMC Musculoskelet Disord. 2016;30(17):193.
18. Kennedy MI, Claes S, Fuso FA, et al. The anterolateral ligament: an anatomic, radiographic, and biomechanical analysis. Am J Sports Med. 2015;43(7):1606–15. https://doi.org/10.1177/0363546515578253.

19. Wytrykowski K, Swider P, Reina N, et al. Cadaveric study comparing the biomechanical properties of grafts used for knee anterolateral ligament reconstruction. Arthroscopy. 2016;32(11):2288–94.
20. Monaco E, Lanzetti RM, Fabbri M, et al. Anterolateral ligament reconstruction with autologous grafting: a biomechanical study. Clin Biomech (Bristol, Avon). 2017;44:99–103.
21. Sugita T, Amis AA. Anatomic and biomechanical study of the lateral collateral and popliteofibular ligaments. Am J Sports Med. 2001;29(4):466–72.
22. Cooper DE, Deng XH, Burstein AL, et al. The strength of the central third patellar tendon graft. A biomechanical study. Am J Sports Med. 1993;21(6):818–23.
23. Muller W. The knee. New York: Springer Verlag; 1983.
24. Hardy A, Ferreira FB, Hunter JC. Segond fracture after anterior cruciate ligament reconstruction. Radiol Case Rep. 2015;4(3):305.
25. Ferretti A, Monaco E, Wolf MR, et al. Surgical treatment of Segond fractures in acute anterior cruciate ligament reconstruction. Orthop J Sports Med. 2017;5(10):2325967117729997.
26. Mazza D, Monaco E, Redler A, et al. Segond fractures involve the anterolateral knee capsule but not the iliotibial band. Arthrosc Sports Med Rehabil. 2021;3(3):e639–43.
27. Ferretti A, Monaco E, Ponzo A, et al. Combined intra-articular and extra-articular reconstruction in anterior cruciate ligament-deficient knee: 25 years later. Arthroscopy. 2016;32(10):2039–47.
28. Guzzini M, Mazza D, Fabbri M, et al. Extra-articular tenodesis combined with an anterior cruciate ligament reconstruction in acute anterior cruciate ligament tear in elite female football players. Int Orthop. 2016;40(10):2091–6.
29. Redler A, Iorio R, Monaco E, et al. Revision anterior cruciate ligament reconstruction with hamstrings and extra-articular tenodesis: a mid- to long-term clinical and radiological study. Arthroscopy. 2018;34(12):3204–13.
30. Yoon KH, Kim JS, Park SY, et al. The influence of segond fracture on outcomes after anterior cruciate ligament reconstruction. Arthroscopy. 2018;34(6):1900–6.

The Unhappy Triad Revisited

6

Andrea Ferretti and Daniele Mazza

The term "unhappy triad" was first used in 1964 by one of the fathers of orthopaedic sports medicine, O'Donoghue [1], and identifies a very serious knee injury affecting the anterior cruciate ligament (ACL), medial collateral ligament (MCL) and medial meniscus, occurring in an estimated 25% of acute athletic knee injuries. According to this feature, the unhappy triad would correspond to an anteromedial rotatory instability (AMRI), according to the classification proposed by Hughston et al. [2]. This pattern of instability is recognized by a positive Lachman test, valgus stress test and due to the involvement of the ACL eventually Jerk test, even if the Jerk test could be difficult to evaluate due to the loss of a valid medial support.

The characterization of this injury, as far as it concerned the involvement of the medial meniscus, was questioned as a result of the advent of arthroscopy. In fact, Shelbourne and Nitz [3] reported a higher prevalence of lateral, rather than medial, meniscal tears, suggesting wider involvement of the lateral compartment than previously reported. Other authors [4–6] later supported the findings of Shelbourne and Nitz.

However, Mueller, in his 1982 book "The Knee: Form, Function, and Ligament Reconstruction" [7], had already addressed this topic, reporting that "during the routine exposure of fresh unhappy triad injuries, we frequently found that they were actually tetrad injuries, the fourth component being a fresh lesion of the anterolateral femorotibial ligament (ALFTL)". The author had already described the ALFTL as a distal portion of the iliotibial tract extending from the linea aspera, just below the femoral attachment of the lateral collateral ligament, to the Gerdy tubercle (See Fig. 2.9, Chap. 2).

More recently, there has been a renewed focus on the anatomy [8–12] and function [13–17] of the structures of the lateral compartment acting as secondary restraints of the ACL in controlling the internal rotation of the tibia. Anatomical

A. Ferretti (✉) · D. Mazza
Orthopaedic Unit, Sant'Andrea University Hospital, La Sapienza University, Rome, Italy

A. Ferretti (ed.), *Anterolateral Rotatory Instability in ACL Deficient Knee*, https://doi.org/10.1007/978-3-031-00115-4_6

descriptions led to the identification of the anterolateral ligament (ALL), considered the main structure of the anterolateral complex, which also includes the deep portion of the iliotibial tract (the so-called capsulo-osseous layer) and the posterior horn of the lateral meniscus.

A possible extensive and simultaneous involvement of the anterolateral compartment, along with the ACL and medial compartment, would change the type of instability, as this pattern of lesions would inevitably result in a combined AMRI and anterolateral rotatory instability (ALRI).

It would therefore be extremely interesting to investigate how often a combined AMRI and ALRI instability occurs in a setting of ACL tears, as they would be surgically addressed accordingly.

In 2014, after a three-month trial, our hospital launched a pilot study aimed to offer to all patients referred to our emergency department with the clinical suspicion of an ACL tear, a dedicated pathway finalized to perform the surgical treatment, whenever needed, within a maximum of two weeks since the initial injury (acute phase). This project was named "two for two" after a similar project that was supported by the NHS to encourage early treatment of femoral neck fractures in the elderly population: two days for femoral neck fractures in elderly individuals and two weeks for ACL tears in younger individuals and the athletic population.

To date, more than 300 consecutive acute ACL reconstructions have been performed, and their clinical and surgical charts were collected and recorded in detail. Patients presenting with a positive Lachman test and positive valgus stress at the initial clinical evaluation were considered possible cases of combined AMRI and ALRI. According to our preoperative protocol, all patients were assessed clinically and radiologically with standard X-ray and 1,5T magnetic resonance imaging (MRI). A clinical evaluation was repeated under anaesthesia, and an evaluation of the severity of the MCL injury was performed, with the aid of a fluoroscope, by a valgus stress test at 30° of flexion (Fig. 6.1).

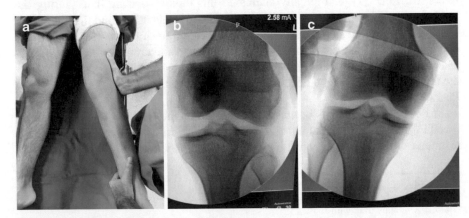

Fig. 6.1 (a) Positive valgus stress at 30° of flexion, (b) Fluoroscopy revealed a level III MCL tear with resulting III-degree instability (opening > 10 mm) as compared with the healthy side (c)

Patients with grade III instability (medial opening of more than 10 mm) underwent open MCL repair, while other MCL injuries were treated conservatively. In all patients, the lateral compartment was surgically addressed, and the anterolateral complex was inspected and surgically treated whenever needed. In the operated patients, the MCL was approached through an incision on the medial side of the knee, and repair of the MCL was performed with absorbable stitches, with the aid of suture anchors whenever required (Figs. 6.2 and 6.3).

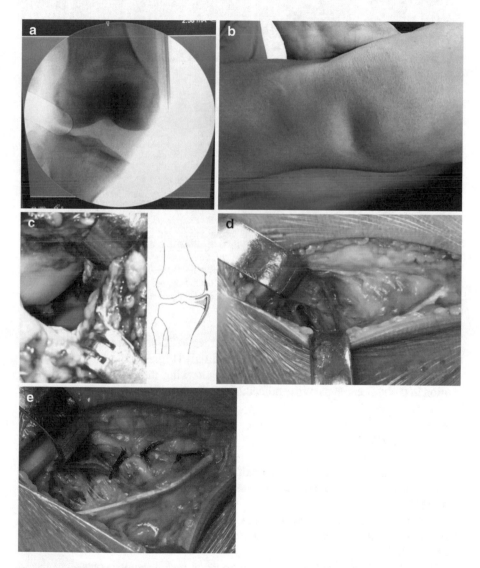

Fig. 6.2 Unhappy triad with III-degree AMRI. (**a**) Fluoroscopy valgus stress test. (**b, c**) The cutaneous depression visible during the valgus stress test ("sulcus sign") indicates a possible invagination of the MCL confirmed at surgery. (**d**) Injury of the anterolateral capsule (type 3, complete). (**e**) Repair/retensioning of the anterolateral ligament and capsule

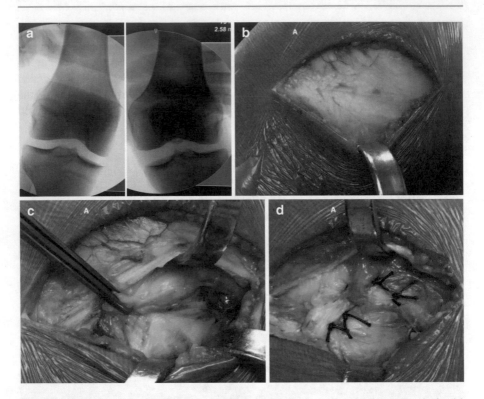

Fig. 6.3 Unhappy triad with II-degree AMRI (opening 5–10 mm), treated conservatively. (**a**) Fluoroscopy revealed a III-level MCL tear with a resulting II-degree instability as compared with the healthy side. (**b**) Fascia lata appeared quite normal. (**c**) Injury of the anterolateral capsule (type 2). (**d**) Repair/retensioning of the anterolateral capsule

In selected cases, the site of the tear of the deep MCL was assessed arthroscopically, and the skin incision was reduced accordingly (Fig. 6.4).

Overconstraint was avoided by repeatedly checking the stability and range of motion in the various steps of the procedure.

6.1   Surgical Findings

The surgical findings refer to a series of eleven cases collected during a period of three years among a consecutive series of 125 patients with acute ACL tears [18].

As a result of fluoroscopy examination, medial compartment was treated conservatively in eight patients (II-degree AMRI) and surgically in three (III-degree AMRI).

The ACL was completely torn in all patients; a medial meniscus tear was found in one patient and treated by partial meniscectomy; lateral meniscus tears were

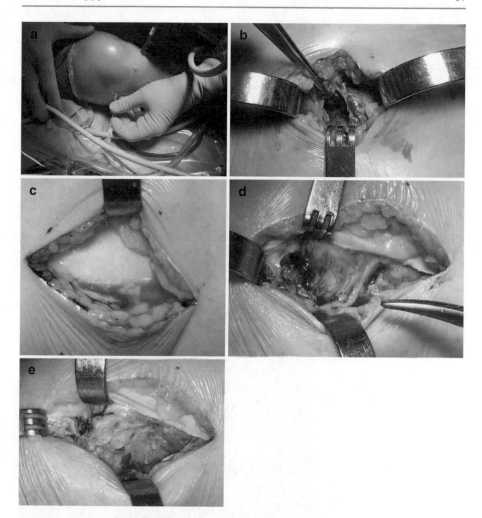

Fig. 6.4 Mini-open repair of MCL in a severe case of unhappy triad. (**a**) Arthroscopically assisted identification of the site of the MCL tear. (**b**) A mini-open approach and repair of the MCL tear. (**c**) Lateral compartment exposure: overflow reveals a possible tear of the anterolateral complex with possible lack of the permeability of the apparently normal fascia lata. (**d**, **e**) The capsule was approached by splitting the fascia lata and a complete tear of the anterolateral ligament (type III lesion) was identified and surgically repaired

found in three patients: surgical repair was performed for two patients while a partial, selective, meniscectomy was performed for one patient. Standard ACL reconstruction with the hamstrings was performed for all patients.

In all cases, the lateral compartment was also inspected through a 5–7 cm long hockey stick incision that was proximal to Gerdy's tubercle. The fascia lata was apparently normal or quite normal in seven cases (Fig. 6.5) and haemorrhagic in 4 cases (Fig. 6.6).

Fig. 6.5 Normal aspect of the fascia lata

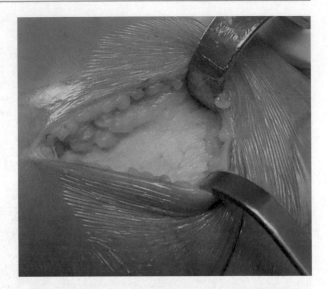

Fig. 6.6 Fascia lata appeared frankly haemorrhagic

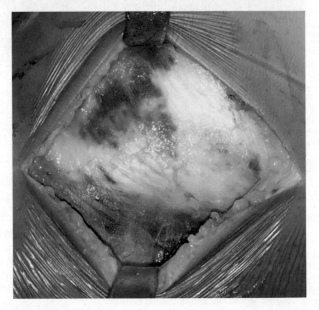

The fascia lata was then longitudinally split to expose the capsule. The anterolateral complex was frankly damaged in all cases: there was one case of a type I lesion, 7 cases of type II lesions (Fig. 6.7), 2 cases of type III lesions (Fig. 6.8) and one case of a type IV lesion (Segond's fracture). All tears were accurately repaired, and the complex was retensioned by plication using absorbable stitches.

At follow-up, in 2 patients, mild valgus stress (+ – –) was found to not affect day life or sports activities. The Lachman test was negative for all patients. The pivot

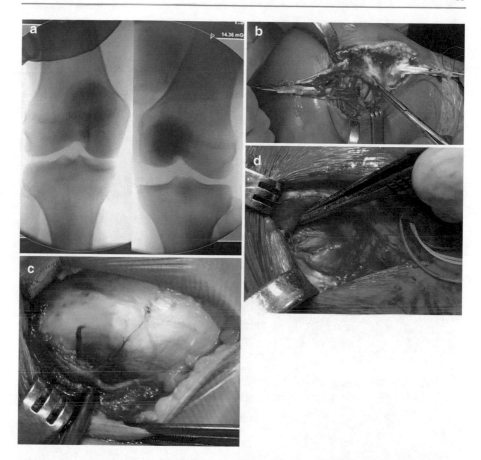

Fig. 6.7 III-degree AMRI (**a**) Fluoroscopy revealed a level III MCL tear with resulting III-degree instability as compared with the healthy side. (**b**) Extensive damage of both superficial MCL (sMCL) and deep MCL (dMCL). (**c**) Fascia lata appeared stretched and haemorrhagic. (**d**) A complete tear of the anterolateral ligament (type II lesion) was identified and surgically repaired

shift test was negative in 9 patients and mildly positive (glide + − −) in 2 patients. There were eight patients with ISAKOS class A and 3 patients with class B with no patients with class C and D. All patients had recovered full ROM.

All patients returned to their preoperative level of activity, including for sports.

The most important finding of our experience as reported here is that the "unhappy triad", as already postulated by Mueller in the early eighties, should be considered a tetrad of injuries, with the fourth component being the concurrent lesion of the anterolateral complex. However, injury to the anterolateral complex could be difficult to diagnose preoperatively, as the lack of valid medial support can sometimes make the pivot shift difficult to elicit.

Indications for the surgical repair of III-level MCL tears are another matter of debate. Many authors recommend conservative treatment [19–22], while others

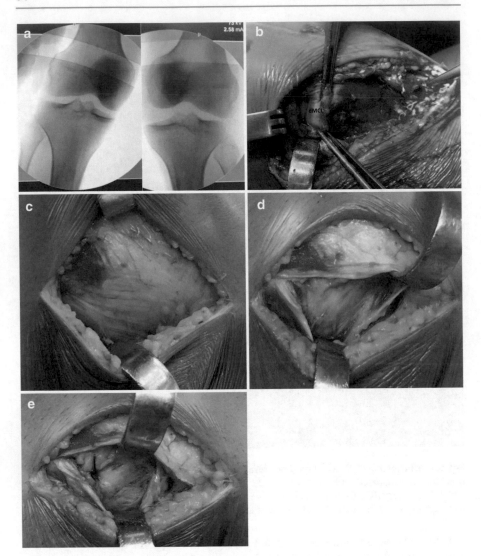

Fig. 6.8 (**a**) Fluoroscopy. (**b**) Complete tear of the deep MCL (dMCL) in its femoro-meniscal band. (**c**) Fascia lata was mildly stretched and haemorrhagic. (**d, e**) Type 2 lesion of the anterolateral complex and its retensioning

suggest surgical treatment [4], either early or delayed, after a few weeks in cases of spontaneous healing failure. This concern could be due to confusion, which still exists among the terms used in the classification of ligament tears and instabilities. In fact, our approach to the surgical treatment of MCL tears is limited to complete tears (level III ligament tears) leading to a III-degree medial instability only, as identified by a medial opening of more than 10 mm through a valgus stress test in mild flexion. While complete medial collateral ligament tears can occur in

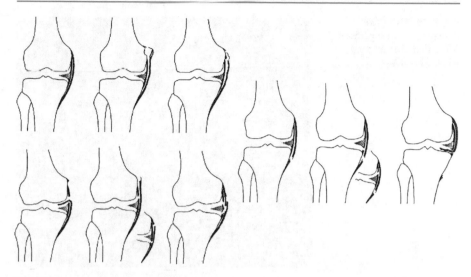

Fig. 6.9 Pattern of injuries involving the MCL according to Muller (Reprinted with permission from: W. Mueller "The Knee" Springer-Verlag, Berlin 1982, pages 148–154)

approximately 25% of all ACL tears, grade III instability occurs in no more than 3% of cases. Our advice to proceed with early surgical treatment of these injuries is justified because tears are more easily recognized and reparable in this acute phase and supported by our clinical results.

In addition to his brilliant intuition in identifying the previously unrecognized fourth element of the unhappy triad, Mueller should also be credited for his excellent description of the pattern of injuries involving the MCL in either its superficial or deep bands (Fig. 6.9).

In our experience, which spans much longer than 7 years and in fact dates back to the early eighties, we have had the chance to observe and successfully repair almost all types of injuries described by Muller (Figs. 6.10, 6.11 and 6.12).

However, the key for the successful surgical treatment of the unhappy triad is not only early repair of medial and lateral structures performed along with intraarticular ACL reconstruction but also accelerated rehabilitation and a strict postoperative check of the progressive recovery of Range of Motion (ROM). As the risk of stiffness and arthrofibrosis is potentially high, all operated patients should be followed from the first postoperative day, carefully observing the basic principle of "maintain the extension and encourage flexion" for rehabilitation. The use of continuous passive motion (CPM) devices should also be considered. In our experience, combined MCL and ACL surgery represents the only indication for the use of CPM devices in post-ACL reconstruction rehabilitation. Despite accurate follow-up of the rehabilitation process, a delay of recovery of the ROM could be occasionally observed, requiring manipulation under anaesthesia. When needed, this procedure should be successfully performed between two or three months postoperatively with any further adverse events.

Fig. 6.10 Extensive damage of both superficial MCL (sMCL) and deep MCL (dMCL)

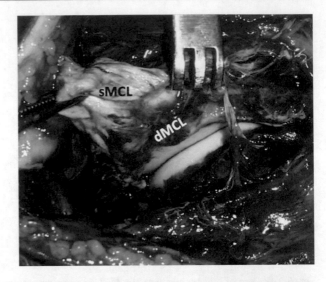

Fig. 6.11 The "floating meniscus": combined of both of meniscofemoral and meniscotibial bands of MCL

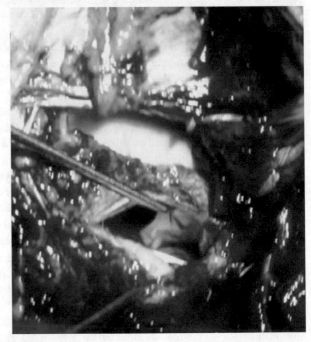

Historically, the unhappy triad has been ascribed to a valgus external rotation mechanism, in which the medial compartment is injured first, followed by a tear of the ACL.

However, this specific mechanism of injury does not explain the different grades of involvement of the MCL or the constant involvement of the anterolateral complex. Therefore, another mechanism of injury should be postulated.

Fig. 6.12 Distal detachment of sMCL

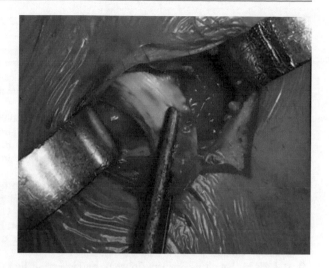

Researchers from the Norwegian Olympic Committee Sports Medicine Center in Oslo published several three-dimensional video analyses on a series of ACL tears that occurred in indoor and outdoor sports as recorded by dedicated video cameras and broadcasted on television [23–25]. They used sophisticated software to analyse, in detail, cases that appeared to be the result of a clear valgus external rotation mechanism. The authors documented that when an ACL tear occurs, in the first 40 ms, the knee is in valgus rotation, but the tibia is put in a forced internal rotation just before the knee eventually collapses in a true valgus external rotation. Therefore, on the basis of this study, in most cases of unhappy triads, the mechanism is initially the same as that described for isolated ACL tears (pivot shift-like mechanism) followed by a sudden collapse of the knee in valgus external rotation. The resulting sequence of injuries is as follows: the ACL tears first, the anterolateral complex tears second (including the ALL and lateral meniscus) and eventually the MCL with the medial meniscus tears. This mechanism of injury, with the late involvement of the MCL, could explain the constant involvement of the anterolateral complex as well as the different degrees of MCL injury severity.

In conclusion, the unhappy triad is in fact a tetrad that includes injuries of the ACL, medial or lateral meniscus, MCL and anterolateral complex. It results from a "two steps" severe knee sprain that, starting from an internal valgus rotation, suddenly turns towards an external valgus rotation. While early ACL reconstruction is advisable in most cases, the surgical repair of the MCL could be needed only in the most severe cases of tears, resulting in a III-degree valgus instability (a medial opening > 10 mm). In the case of MCL repairs, surgeons should pay close attention to postoperative rehabilitation, avoiding the risk of stiffness and arthrofibrosis and possibly requiring manipulation under anaesthesia.

References

1. O'donoghue D. The unhappy triad: etiology, diagnosis and treatment. Am J Orthop. 1964;6:242–7.
2. Hughston JC, Andrews JR, Cross MJ, Moschi A. Classification of knee ligament instabilities. Part I. The medial compartment and cruciate ligaments. J Bone Joint Surg Am. 1976;58(2):159–72.
3. Shelbourne KD, Nitz PA. The O'Donoghue triad revisited. Combined knee injuries involving anterior cruciate and medial collateral ligament tears. Am J Sports Med. 1991;19(5):474–7.
4. Barber FA. What is the terrible triad? Arthroscopy. 1992;8(1):19–22.
5. Dacombe PJ. Shelbourne's update of the O'Donoghue knee triad in a 17-year-old male Rugby player. BMJ Case Rep. 2013;23:2013.
6. Mansori AE, Lording T, Schneider A, Dumas R, Servien E, Lustig S. Incidence and patterns of meniscal tears accompanying the anterior cruciate ligament injury: possible local and generalized risk factors. Int Orthop. 2018;42(9):2113–21.
7. Müller W. The knee: form, function and ligament reconstruction. Berlin: Springer-Verlag; 1982.
8. Claes S, Vereecke E, Maes M, Victor J, Verdonk P, Bellemans J. Anatomy of the anterolateral ligament of the knee. J Anat. 2013;223(4):321–8.
9. Daggett M, Busch K, Sonnery-Cottet B. Surgical dissection of the anterolateral ligament. Arthrosc Tech. 2016;5(1):e185-8.
10. Daggett M, Ockuly AC, Cullen M, Busch K, Lutz C, Imbert P, Sonnery-Cottet B. Femoral origin of the anterolateral ligament: an anatomic analysis. Arthroscopy. 2015;32(5):835–41.
11. Goncharov EN, Koval OA, Bezuglov EN, Goncharov NG. Anatomical features and significance of the anterolateral ligament of the knee. Int Orthop. 2018;42(12):2859–64.
12. Helito CP, Demange MK, Bonadio MB, Tírico LE, Gobbi RG, Pécora JR, Camanho GL. Anatomy and histology of the knee anterolateral ligament. Orthop J Sports Med. 2013;9(1):7.
13. Ferretti A, Monaco E, Fabbri M, Maestri B, De Carli A. Prevalence and classification of injuries of anterolateral complex in acute anterior cruciate ligament tears. Arthroscopy. 2017;33(1):147–54.
14. Rasmussen MT, Nitri M, Williams BT, Moulton SG, Cruz RS, Dornan GJ, Goldsmith MT, LaPrade RF. An in vitro robotic assessment of the anterolateral ligament, part 1: secondary role of the anterolateral ligament in the setting of an anterior cruciate ligament injury. Am J Sports Med. 2016;44(3):585–92.
15. Sonnery-Cottet B, Lutz C, Daggett M, Dalmay F, Freychet B, Niglis L, Imbert P. The involvement of the anterolateral ligament in rotational control of the knee. Am J Sports Med. 2016;44(5):1209–14.
16. Sonnery-Cottet B, Saithna A, Cavalier M, Kajetanek C, Temponi EF, Daggett M, Helito CP, Thaunat M. Anterolateral ligament reconstruction is associated with significantly reduced ACL graft rupture rates at a minimum follow-up of 2 years: a prospective comparative study of 502 patients from the SANTI group. Am J Sports Med. 2017;45(7):1547–57.
17. Sonnery-Cottet B, Thaunat M, Freychet B, Pupim BH, Murphy CG, Claes S. Outcome of a combined anterior cruciate ligament and anterolateral ligament reconstruction technique with a minimum 2-year follow-up. Am J Sports Med. 2015;43(7):1598–605.
18. Ferretti A, Monaco E, Ponzo A, Dagget M, Guzzini M, Mazza D, Redler A, Conteduca F. The unhappy triad of the knee re-revisited. Int Orthop. 2019;43(1):223–8.
19. Ballmer P, Ballmer F, Jakob R. Reconstruction of the anterior cruciate ligament alone in the treatment of a combined instability with complete rupture of the medial collateral ligament. Arch Orthop Trauma Surg. 1991;110:139–41.
20. Hillard-Sembell D, Daniel DM, Stone ML, Dobson BE, Fithian DC. Combined injuries of the anterior cruciate and medial collateral ligaments of the knee. Effect of treatment on stability and function of the joint*. J Bone Joint Surg. 1996;78:169–76.

21. Millett PJ, Pennock AT, Sterett WI, Steadman JR. Early ACL reconstruction in combined ACLMCL injuries. J Knee Surg. 2004;17:94–8.
22. Shelbourne KD, Porter DA. Anterior cruciate ligament-medial collateral ligament injury: Nonoperative management of medial collateral ligament tears with anterior cruciate ligament reconstruction A preliminary report. Am J Sports Med. 1992;20:283–6.
23. Fuller CW, Ekstrand J, Junge A, Andersen TE, Bahr R, Dvorak J, Hägglund M, McCrory P, Meeuwisse WH. Consensus statement on injury definitions and data collection procedures in studies of football (soccer) injuries. Scand J Med Sci Sports. 2006;16(2):83–92.
24. Koga H, Bahr R, MyklebustG EL, Grund T, Krosshaug T. Estimating anterior tibial translation from model-based image-matching of a noncontactanterior cruciate ligament injury in professional football: a case report. Clin J Sport Med. 2011;21(3):271–4.
25. Olsen OE, Myklebust G, Engebretsen L, Bahr R. Injury mechanisms for anterior cruciate ligament injuries in team handball: a systematic video analysis. Am J Sports Med. 2004;32(4):1002–12.

Mechanism of Injury of ACL Tears

7

Angelo De Carli, Andrea Ferretti, and Barbara Maestri

The close correlation between the traumatic mechanism and the site of ligamentous damage has always been considered an important factor that eventually contributes to a reliable diagnosis of knee sprains.

Previous biomechanical, laboratory and video analytic studies [1–12] as well as clinical observations have led to the assessment that the traumatic mechanisms most frequently involved in knee ligament injuries are represented by:

- Valgus and external rotation
- Varus and internal rotation
- Anterior to posterior
- Hyperextension
- Complex trauma that usually results in multiligamentous injuries

Anterior cruciate ligament (ACL) tears are usually referred to as either valgus and external rotation or varus and internal rotation traumatic mechanisms.

Injuries less frequently occur due to trauma in hyperextension (Fig. 7.1) (guillotine mechanism against the roof of the intercondylar notch, Fig. 8.1, Chap. 8) or a violent force anteriorly displacing the proximal extremity of the tibia, eventually produced by a sudden contraction of the quadriceps on a hyperflexed knee (Fig. 7.2). The latter mechanism is considered typical of skiing injuries in the act of resuming the standing position from squatting. Both hyperflexion and hyperextension

A. De Carli (✉) · A. Ferretti · B. Maestri
Orthopaedic Unit, Sant'Andrea University Hospital, La Sapienza University, Rome, Rome, Italy

Fig. 7.1 Hyperextension mechanism

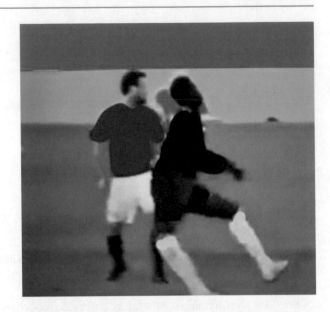

Fig. 7.2 Hyperflexion mechanism

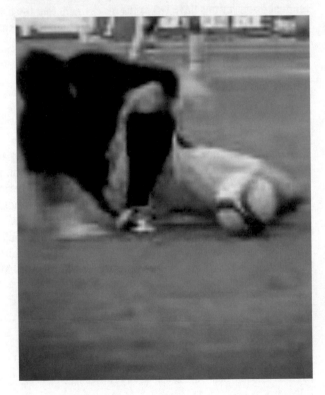

Fig. 7.3 Valgus external
rotation mechanism

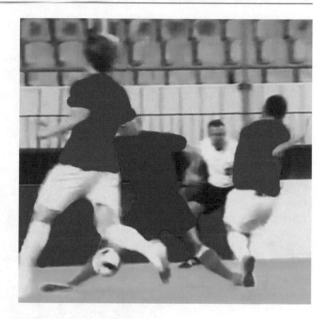

mechanisms would be likely to result in a true isolated lesion of the ACL, as they are
not associated with any rotational torque.

However, the most common mechanism of injury of ACL tears includes sudden
and often violent rotational stress.

In forced valgus and external rotation (Fig. 7.3), the first structure that is stretched
and eventually torn is the medial collateral ligament (MCL) in its superficial and
deep layer; later, the ACL itself is eventually involved, with anteromedial rotatory
instability (AMRI) occurring as a result (Fig. 7.4).

On the other hand, in the varus and internal rotation mechanism (Fig. 7.5), the
first ligament involved is the ACL, followed by the anterolateral complex with an
anterolateral rotatory instability (ALRI) occurring as a result [13–14] (Fig. 7.6).

At the beginning of my professional activity, as a resident, I collected patients'
clinical histories in an attempt to recognize the traumatic mechanism to determine
the site of possible ligamentous damage; I remember myself frequently recording
the patients' descriptions of traumas in valgus external rotation. Very often, this history did not match the kind of instability that was actually observed as a result of
physical examinations, where while the Lachman or pivot shift tests were positive,
the valgus stress test was fully negative.

This mismatch between the traumatic mechanism (valgus and external rotation),
the actual site of the ligamentous damage, ACL and anterolateral ligament (ALL)
and the related ALRI has been an unsolved problem for many years, at least in relation to my personal evaluations and clinical knowledge.

Fig. 7.4 Valgus external
rotation

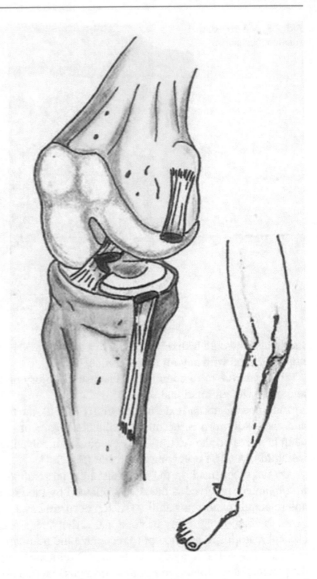

Even the video analysis of some recorded television footage of many cases of
ACL injuries in professional footballers from various international leagues was not
able to better clarify this issue.

Recently, thanks to the collaboration with the Match Analysis Department of the
Italian Football Association, led by Antonio Gagliardi and Filippo Lorenzon, which
has access to the largest database of recorded football matches of all the major
European National Leagues, we conducted a detailed video analysis of 128 ACL
injuries in European football players, which could be worthy of reporting in detail
[2]. The aim of this study was to investigate all the circumstances of ACL tears,
including the mechanism of injuries occurring in high-level football players in

Fig. 7.5 Varus internal rotation mechanism

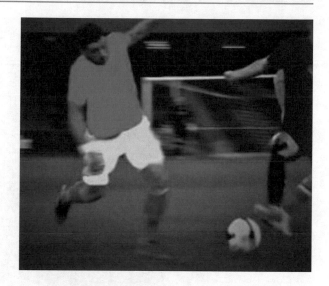

Fig. 7.6 Varus internal rotation

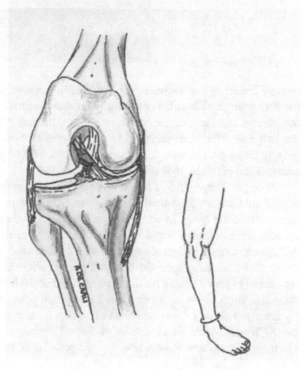

official matches. The main finding of the study was that most ACL tears (72%) occurred in the first half (45 min) of the game, with a peak (52%) in the first 30 minutes. These figures, in addition to downsizing the role of fatigue in the pathogenesis of ACL tears, highlight the importance of the speed of the game, which is

Fig. 7.7 Deceleration
with posterior centre of
gravity

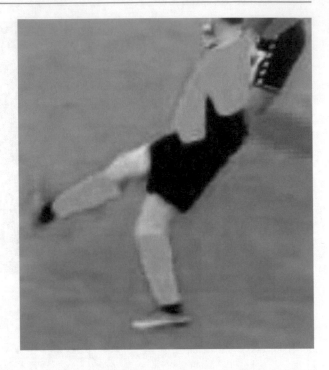

usually higher at the beginning of the match. Another interesting finding includes
the low number of injuries resulting from direct trauma (28%). Moreover, 52% of
the players were in a defensive phase, 38% were engaged in an attempt to recover
the ball and 59% were engaged in high-speed motion. Interestingly, 47% of the
players had a posterior centre of gravity at the time of injury, which occurred in a
deceleration phase in 36% of cases (Fig. 7.7).

While goalkeepers had a lower risk of injury, defenders, midfielders and attack-
ers did not have any statistically significant difference in their rate of tears. Based on
the results of the study, by analysing all the recorded data, we speculated that deceleration, landing from a jump and a sudden change of direction, mostly involved in
ACL tears, require a fast, strong and well-coordinated eccentric contraction of the
lower limb muscles, especially the quadriceps. When an athlete loses neuromuscu-
lar control in performing a required adjustment of the body and knee balance, movement that stresses the joint occurs at a nonreturn point, and an ACL tear can occur.
By deeply analysing the mechanism of injury, it seemed that in most cases (>62%),
the ACL tears were the result of a forced valgus external rotation movement.
Therefore, a mismatch between the supposed mechanism of injury, suggesting
anteromedial instability, and the actual surgical and clinical findings, with a higher
prevalence of anterolateral instability, persisted.

A convincing explanation for this apparent contradiction was recently provided
to us by a series of works published by the Norwegian Sports Medicine Olympic
Center research team in Oslo.

These authors developed very sophisticated software [7] for the video analysis of knee trauma that allows, through the use of high-definition cameras, the superimposition of the skeleton on the surface of the body (in this case, the femur and tibia) to observe the reciprocal movements of joint surfaces in real time.

The most accurate 3D reconstruction of traumatic movement is carried out thanks to various video cameras and requires considerable time and specific competence and experience, but the resulting reliability is high.

The first application of this new technology was carried out with players of an indoor sport (handball) whose actions are more easily investigated, as the distance from the cameras to the players is lower and more reproducible. By analysing the mechanism of injuries of 10 players who sustained a surgically confirmed ACL tear while playing handball, the software provided a sequence of images allowing us to exactly frame the knee at the exact time when the ACL tear occurred [6].

At the moment of rupture, which occurs within approximately 40 milliseconds, the knee is actually posed in valgus and slight flexion, but the tibia rotates internally. Only afterwards, a few milliseconds later did the tibia "counterrotate" externally (Table 7.1).

Table 7.1 Time sequences of 10 cases with knee rotation angles in degrees (°). The thick black line indicates the mean with the 95% confidence interval (shown in the grey area). Time 0 is the initial condition, and the black vertical line indicates the time of 40 milliseconds after the initial condition. Ext rotation: external rotation; *Int.* rotation: internal rotation. Koga H, AJSM 2010 [6]

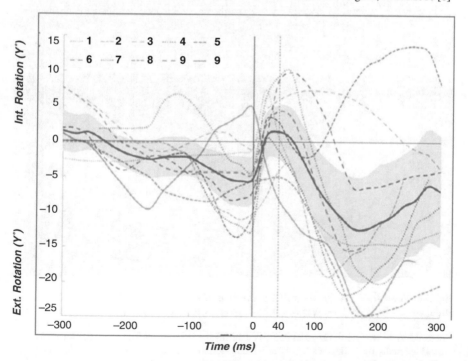

Much more complicated is the video-analytical study of the traumas of outdoor sports such as football. However, the same technology was successfully used to investigate a very popular knee injury, broadcast worldwide, that occurred for one of the most distinguished players of the England National Team, whose ACL was torn during an official match against Sweden. The analysis of this injury, which occurred live, shown in all reviews and slow-motion pictures as a typical valgus external rotation sprain with possible involvement of both the ACL and MCL, was the subject of a case report later published by the same group [5]. In fact, by reviewing the injury using the dedicated software, in the first 30 milliseconds (Fig. 7.8), while the knee was in a forced valgus and mild flexion, the knee was externally rotated by 11 degrees at initial contact (the first frame where the foot contacted the ground before the injury) (Fig. 7.8a); then, the tibia quickly internally rotated by 21

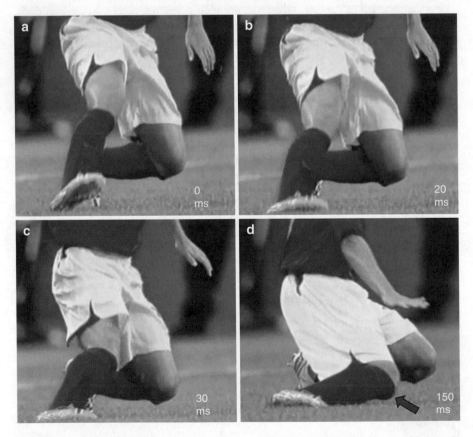

Fig. 7.8 Video frames of the footballer at the time of knee trauma resulting in an ACL tear. At initial contact (IC), the knee was flexed 35 degrees, with an external rotation of 11 degrees and neutral abduction angle (**a**). Anterior tibial translation started to occur 20 milliseconds after the IC, where the knee was the most extended (**b**). During the first 30 milliseconds, the knee abruptly rotated internally by 21 degrees (**c**). After 30 milliseconds, the knee abduction angle had increased by 21 degrees and then changed its direction to external rotation (**d**)

degrees during the first 30 milliseconds (Fig. 7.8b); soon thereafter, the tibia counter-rotated (Fig. 7.8c) and the knee finally collapsed in valgus and external rotation (Fig. 7.8d).

As a result, as soon as the ACL fails, the secondary restraints of tibial internal rotation in the anterolateral compartment could become stretched and eventually injured, often aggravating the ALRI [14, 15]. Only in the most severe sprains, as a consequence of the eventual valgus external rotation collapse, is the medial compartment involved, resulting in the so-called "unhappy triad" [16].

It is likely that this complex and very fast mechanism is not perceived by the patient, who usually only remember valgus stress along with an abnormal sudden movement leading to the knee giving way and instability.

The mechanism of injury has also been indirectly investigated by radiologists who tried to recognize the movement that possibly leads to ACL tears by analysing the location of bone bruises, as revealed by magnetic resonance imaging (MRI) performed for acute tears. In fact, as reported by some authors [17–19], the location of bone bruises, which can occur at the posterolateral tibial plateau, at the anterolateral femoral condyle or at both locations (Fig. 7.9a, b, c), leads to the conclusion that forced internal rotation of the tibia actually occurs, causing the posterolateral tibial plateau to hit against the anterolateral femoral condyle.

In this way, a violent impact of the anterolateral condyle over the posterolateral tibial plateau is likely to occur, possibly resulting in an "occult fracture" (bone bruise).

In conclusion, ACL injuries are mostly due to forced movement in valgus and internal rotation, a very unnatural traumatic mechanism. Patients are usually unable to reliably describe the mechanism of injury, as they often only remember the valgus sprain.

What the detailed video analysis provided by the Norwegian researchers and the MRI studies on bone bruises clearly suggested is a brilliant idea that seems obvious in retrospect: ACL tears are mostly the result of a forced pivot shift-like mechanism

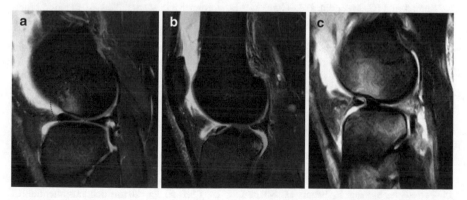

Fig. 7.9 Characteristic bone bruising observed in acute ACL tears; at the anterolateral femoral condyle (**a**), at the posterolateral tibial plateau (**b**) and at both the anterolateral femoral condyle and posterolateral tibial plateau (**c**)

(valgus internal rotation in mild flexion), which are so well reproduced (and often recognized as unhappily familiar by the patient) by rotational laxity tests [16].

References

1. Bere T, Mok KM, Koga H, Krosshaug T, Nordsletten L, Bahr R. Kinematics of anterior cruciate ligament ruptures in World Cup alpine skiing: 2 case reports of the slip-catch mechanism. Am J Sports Med. 2013;41(5):1067–73.
2. De Carli A, Koverech G, Gaj E, Marzilli F, Fantoni F, Liberati Petrucci G, Lorenzon F, Ferretti A. Anterior cruciate ligament injury in elite football players: video analysis of 128 cases. J Sports Med Phys Fitness. 2022;62(2):222–8. https://doi.org/10.23736/S0022-4707.21.11230-7. Epub 2021 Jun 1. PMID: 34080810.
3. Grassi A, Smiley SP, Roberti di Sarsina T, Signorelli C, Marcheggiani Muccioli GM, Bondi A, et al. Mechanisms and situations of anterior cruciate ligament injuries in professional male soccer players: a YouTube-based video analysis. Eur J Orthop Surg Traumatol. 2017;27(7):967–81.
4. Johnston JT, Mandelbaum BR, Schub D, Rodeo SA, Matava MJ, Silvers-Granelli HJ, et al. Video analysis of anterior cruciate ligament tears in professional american football athletes. Am J Sports Med. 2018;46(4):862–8.
5. Koga H, Bahr R, Myklebust G, Engebretsen L, Grund T, Krosshaug T. Estimating anterior tibial translation from model-based image-matching of a noncontact anterior cruciate ligament injury in professional football: a case report. Clin J Sport Med. 2011;21(3):271–4.
6. Koga H, Nakamae A, Shima Y, Iwasa J, Myklebust G, Engebretsen L, et al. Mechanisms for noncontact anterior cruciate ligament injuries: knee joint kinematics in 10 injury situations from female team handball and basketball. Am J Sports Med. 2010;38(11):2218–25.
7. Krosshang T, Slauterbeck JR, Engebretsen L, Bahr R. Biomechanical analysis of anterior cruciate ligament injury mechanisms: three-dimensional motion reconstruction from video sequences. Scand J Med Sci Sports. 2007;17(5):508–19.
8. Montgomery C, Blackburn J, Withers D, Tierney G, Moran C, Simms C. Mechanisms of ACL injury in professional rugby union: a systematic video analysis of 36 cases. Br J Sports Med. 2018;52(15):994–1001.
9. Olsen OE, Myklebust G, Engebretsen L, Bahr R. Injury mechanisms for anterior cruciate ligament injuries in team handball: a systematic video analysis. Am J Sports Med. 2004;32(4):1002–12.
10. Stuelcken MC, Mellifont DB, Gorman AD, Sayers MG. Mechanisms of anterior cruciate ligament injuries in elite women's netball: a systematic videoanalysis. J Sports Sci. 2016;34(16):1516–22.
11. Teitz CC. Video analysis of ACL injuries. In: Griffin LY, editor. Prevention of noncontact ACL injuries. Rosemont: American Academy of Orthopaedic Surgeons; 2001. p. 87–92.
12. Waldén M, Krosshaug T, Bjørneboe J, Andersen TE, Faul O, Hägglund M. Three distinct mechanisms predominate in non-contact anterior cruciate ligament injuries in male professional football players: a systematic video analysis of 39 cases. Br J Sports Med. 2015;49(22):1452–60.
13. Shelbourne KD, Nitz PA. The O'Donoghue triad revisited. Combined knee injuries involving anterior cruciate and medial collateral ligament tears. Am J Sports Med Sep-Oct. 1991;19(5):474–7.
14. Sonnery-Cottet B, Lutz C, Daggett M, Dalmay F, Freychet B, Niglis L, ImbertP. The involvement of the anterolateral ligament in rotational control of the knee. Am J Sports Med. 2016;44(5):1209–14.
15. Ferretti A, Monaco E, Fabbri M, Maestri B, De Carli A. Prevalence and classification of injuries of anterolateral complex in acute anterior cruciate ligament tears. Arthroscopy. 2017;33(1):147–54.

16. Ferretti A, Monaco E, Ponzo A, Dagget M, Guzzini M, Mazza D, et al. The unhappy triad of the knee re-revisited. Int Orthop. 2019;43(1):223–8.
17. Ferretti A, Monaco E, Redler A, Argento G, De Carli A, Saithna A, et al. High prevalence of anterolateral ligament abnormalities on MRI in knees with acute anterior cruciate ligament injuries: a case-control series from the SANTI Study Group. Orthop J Sports Med. 2019;7(6):2325967119852916.
18. Kim SY, Spritzer CE, Utturkar GM, Toth AP, Garrett WE, DeFrate LE. Knee kinematics during noncontact anterior cruciate ligament injury as determined from bone Bruise location. Am J Sports Med. 2015;43(10):2515–21.
19. Patel SA, Hageman J, Quatman CE, Wordeman SC, Hewett TE. Prevalence and location of bone bruises associated with anterior cruciate ligament injury and implications for mechanism of injury: a systematic review. Sports Med. 2014;44(2):281–93.

Diagnostics in ACL-Deficient Knee

8

Andrea Ferretti, Barbara Maestri, and Ferdinando Iannotti

It is well accepted that the diagnosis of an anterior cruciate ligament (ACL) injury is mainly clinical, with history and physical examination being of the upmost importance. However, a doctor's experience and confidence in performing ligament laxity tests could significantly increase diagnostic accuracy.

The mechanism of injury should be the first factor that is investigated, as the ACL usually tears as a result of a sudden cutting or pivoting movement while running, especially in the deceleration phase, as well as when landing from a jump when the body is unbalanced. Extreme hyperextension (Fig. 8.1) and forced quadriceps contraction (antero-posterior shift mechanism), which require a patient to resume a standing position from a squat or to prevent a backwards fall, have also been reported to cause ACL tears. Another possible mechanism was postulated by evaluating an ACL injury in a skier [1]. The centrality of the forwards rotational acceleration of the tibia caused by the ski boot during landing after a jump in a more or less backwards position without falling was noted. This acceleration caused a compensatory contraction of the quadriceps, followed by an antero-posterior displacement of the femur on the tibia, which caused the ACL injury (see Chap. 7).

However, when a mechanism other than rotation is involved, an isolated ACL tear is more likely to occur, because the secondary restraints are usually less compromised.

In the case of ACL tears, patients often report a sensation of displacement or unnatural movement of the knee. Instead, the sensation of the knee giving way can occur immediately or a few minutes later, as the result of a new cutting movement, when the athlete attempts to resume sports activity. In the case of ACL tears, haemarthrosis usually develops within minutes or a few hours. When effusion later appears, two or more days after trauma, it can be related to hydrarthrosis, which is usually due to less severe injury.

A. Ferretti (✉) · B. Maestri · F. Iannotti
Orthopaedic Unit, Sant'Andrea University Hospital, La Sapienza University, Rome, Italy

© The Author(s), under exclusive license to Springer Nature
Switzerland AG 2022
A. Ferretti (ed.), *Anterolateral Rotatory Instability in ACL Deficient Knee*,
https://doi.org/10.1007/978-3-031-00115-4_8

Fig. 8.1 ACL rupture in extreme hyperextension

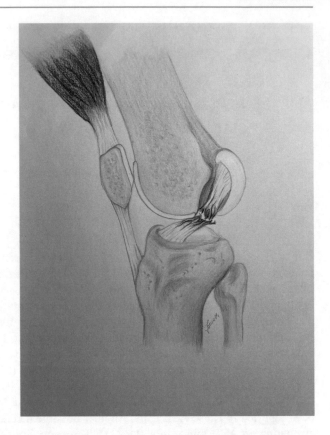

The Lachman test is the most important test for the diagnosis of ACL injuries. In fact, by comparing the correlation of operative findings with other popular clinical tests for anterior and medial instability, it was recognized that the Lachman test is a simple, reliable, and reproducible method for demonstrating anterior cruciate ligament deficiency [2]. Even though its accuracy has been reported to be as high as 100%, more reliable studies have reported a sensitivity of 87% and specificity of 93% [3]. In addition to its extreme accuracy, it can be performed for almost any condition immediately after the injury, even with a swollen and painful knee.

In the Lachman test, the patient is positioned supine with the traumatized knee flexed at 25–35°. The leg is slightly externally rotated to relax the iliotibial band. The examiner then stabilizes the distal femur with one hand and grabs the proximal tibia with the other hand. Anterior force is applied to the tibia in an attempt to subluxate it forwards while keeping the femur stabilized (Figs. 8.2 and 8.3)

ACL deficiency causes anterior tibial translation, which is greater than that in a contralateral healthy knee. The amount of antero-posterior (AP) laxity of the knee resulting from an ACL tear is classified into three degrees of severity. Grade I indicates mild stability, with an increased anterior tibial translation up to 5 mm. Grade II indicates a moderate instability with anterior tibial translation from 6 to 10 mm. Grade III indicates a serious injury with tibial translation greater than 10 mm [4].

Fig. 8.2 The Lachman test

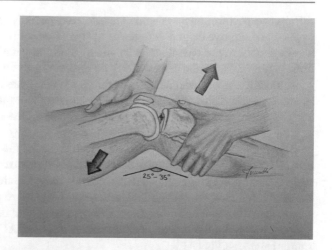

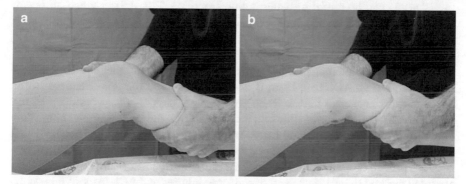

Fig. 8.3 Clinical Lachman test. (**a**) The examiner stabilizes the distal femur with one hand and grabs the proximal tibia with the other hand. (**b**) Anterior force is applied to the tibia in an attempt to subluxate it forwards

Arthrometers have been introduced to more accurately measure the amount of anterior tibial displacement, the most popular being the KT 1000 and 2000 and Rolimeter. Only in a few cases can Lachman test results be difficult to evaluate due to large thighs, hypertrophic quadriceps, a very contracted knee, previous knee injuries, or previous ipsilateral or contralateral reconstructions.

The main limitation of the Lachman test is that it only evaluates the anterior translation of the tibia.

More accurate and dynamic tests, such as the pivot shift and jerk tests, specifically used to evaluate rotational laxity, can give a more comprehensive feature of the overall instability resulting from an ACL tear. In fact, these tests reproduce the traumatic mechanism that is responsible for most ACL injuries. Currently, there is a broad consensus in the scientific community on their qualitative and quantitative grading (+glide, ++ clunk, +++ subluxation). The main limitation of these dynamic tests is their unreliability in acute cases due to swelling, pain, and muscular contraction usually occurring a few hours after the injury, when the dynamic tests are very difficult to perform and evaluate. Therefore, especially in acute and problematic cases, the definitive diagnosis in terms of the extent of rotational instability can be assessed only in the operating room when, with the patient under anaesthesia, the knee is fully relaxed and can carefully be re-examined.

Although a careful and reliable diagnosis of ACL tears can be assessed clinically in most cases and proper treatment can be planned accordingly, in common practice, a series of imaging techniques are used to support a physician in their final evaluation and diagnosis.

Standard X-ray tests are commonly performed in the emergency unit and the results are usually negative and not proven. Only rare proximal bony detachment, as well as tibial spine avulsion, which can be observed in children and adolescents, can be easily detected by standard X-rays (Fig. 8.4). Moreover, Segond's fractures, which actually represent a tibial avulsion of the anterolateral ligament (ALL), are truly considered reliable, indirect radiological signs of ACL tears and anterolateral rotational instability (ALRI).

CT scans can be useful to better define fractures (Fig. 8.5) or when an occult fracture is suspected but are much less accurate in detecting soft tissue injuries such as ACL and ALL tears.

Therefore, magnetic resonance imaging (MRI) alone is able to provide a comprehensive and detailed picture of injuries of ligaments and other soft tissues possibly related to an ACL tear. Even if MRI is considered the gold standard in the instrumental diagnosis of ACL tears, we strongly support the superiority of the clinical findings in a proper assessment of instability and treatment planning. This is even more important in acute cases, when MRI is considered less accurate and promptness in decision-making can be a crucial factor for the outcome of the treatment. However, despite its limitations, MRI remains the most commonly used and accepted method to investigate soft tissue knee injuries and ACL tears. While ACL-related images have been widely described and are usually easily interpreted by

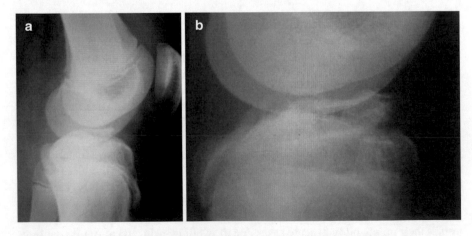

Fig. 8.4 In figures (**a**) and (**b**) X-rays in lateral view show tibial spine avulsion

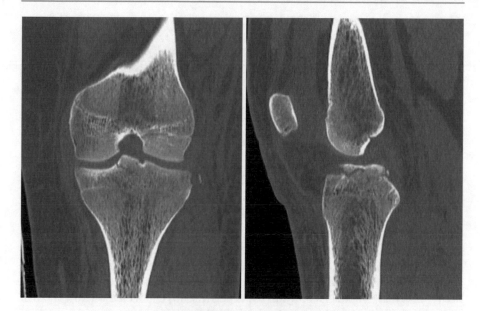

Fig. 8.5 TC scan showing tibial spine fracture and Segond's fracture

Fig. 8.6 Sagittal 1.5 T1 magnetic resonance imaging scans of ACL tears

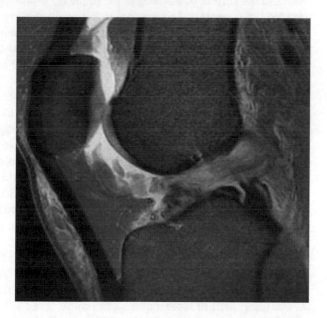

radiologists and orthopaedic surgeons (Fig. 8.6), little is known about the imaging of secondary restraints and anterolateral structures.

Ultrasonography (US) is probably the first and most commonly used instrumental method to investigate secondary restraints and ALL. Orthopaedists, more than radiologists, have used ultrasounds to investigate the normal and pathological

Fig. 8.7 The lateral structures of the knee were used as anatomic landmarks at 35° of flexion. Legend: 1—Gerdy's tubercle; 2—Lateral femoral epicondyle; 3—Anterolateral ligament; 4—joint line

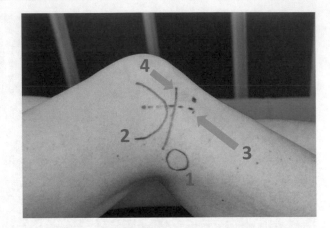

anatomy of the anterolateral complex. This is because this diagnostic tool can be used independently and directly for a patient along with a medical check. In fact, when properly used, ultrasounds can adequately visualize the anterolateral ligament in a reliable and reproducible way. In our experience [5] conducted with a sample of 80 healthy patients, the ALL was clearly visible in a large percentage of the patients, thanks to the correct positioning of the probe by following some simple rules. The anterolateral capsule and ligament were recognized using US in 93.8% (150 out of 160) and 92.5% (148 out of 160) of the knees by Examiner 1 and Examiner 2, respectively, and an appropriate technical procedure was described for its recognition: 30–35° of knee flexion was used after all possible landmarks were identified (Figs. 8.7 and 8.8).

The iliotibial band was used as the first targeting point in all our evaluations. In fact, the ALL distal tract, running between the body of the lateral meniscus and its tibial insertion, is easier to identify once it has been distinguished from the iliotibial band. The distal part of the ALL appears as a hyperechoic band, and the LIGA (lateral inferior geniculate artery) can be used as an easy second anatomical reference landmark. The ALL proximal band seems to be difficult to recognize in some cases, as this band could always be thinner. Once the ALL is identified, its proximal end can also be recognized above the popliteal fossa. Anisotropy artefacts may reduce the echogenicity of the ALL at the middle tract of the proximal band (Figs. 8.9 and 8.10).

Klos et al. [6] used ultrasounds to evaluate Segond's fractures and Segond-like injuries. The most significant finding of the Klos study was a higher prevalence of Segond's fractures identified by ultrasound compared to fractures reported in earlier studies using MRI or radiographs. In his study, 25 of 87 (29%) patients with acute ACL injuries presented an US detectable Segond's fracture or ligament avulsion. By US, the prevalence of Segond's-like injuries was four times higher than the 3–6% diagnosed with MRI by several authors [7–10] and three times higher than the 9% diagnosed with radiography, as reported by Hess et al. [11]. Dynamic ultrasound should be considered an additional imaging modality in acute knee injury diagnosis.

Fig. 8.8 Positioning of a patient for optimal visualization of the ALL: the patient in lateral decubitus on the opposite hip, with knee flexion of 30°–35° and slight internal rotation

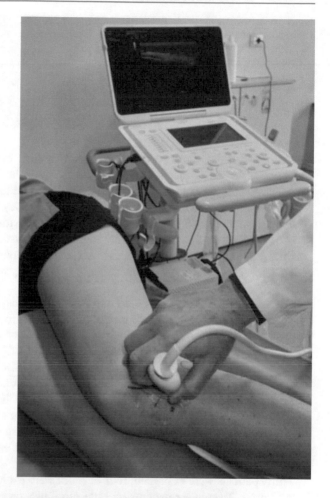

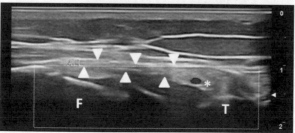

Fig. 8.9 US longitudinal image showing the ALL (arrowheads) as a thin hyperechoic structure running between the lateral femoral condyle and above the popliteal fossa and popliteal tendon. Anisotropy artefacts slightly diminish the echogenicity of the ALL at the middle tract of the proximal band. Legend: F, lateral femoral condyle; T, anterolateral margin of the tibia. Asterisks indicate the LIGA, which can be used as a reference landmark

Fig. 8.10 Longitudinal
US detection of a complete
ALL tear close to its tibial
insertion (Type 3 ALL
injury). Legend: F, lateral
femoral condyle; T,
anterolateral margin of the
tibia

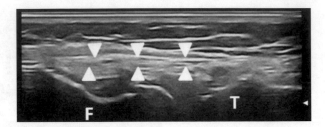

Cavaignac et al. [12] proposed a technique that starts from the localization of the tibial end of the ALL, thanks to the identification of the lateral inferior genicular artery. Eventual lack of tension of the ALL can be identified by the knee internally rotating, therefore recognizing its injury and/or deficiency.

In a recent study by Shekari et al. with 198 patients with ACL tears, 110 (55.6%) had an associated ALL injury that was detected by ultrasound [13].

However, ultrasound is not normally used in knee sprain patients with suspected ACL injuries, and its reliability is considered to be highly related to the ability of the examiner.

Therefore, MRI is the gold standard in radiological diagnostics of a knee with an ACL deficiency and associated injuries of secondary restraints, whose role has recently been emphasized by clinicians. The interest of radiologists has recently switched to investigating the anterolateral complex (ALC) as it appears in MRI.

To better understand ALC features provided by MRI in normal and injured knees, we performed several studies that are worthy of brief report here.

The purpose of the first studies [14] was to describe the anatomy of the ALL of the knee as it appears on a 1.5 Tesla (T) MRI in a series of young patients without reported previous knee injuries. The hypothesis of the study was that the ALL is a distinct structure of the anterolateral capsule that can be easily identified using 1.5-mm slice thickness MRI.

Thirty patients were examined; four of them were excluded because of previous knee injuries. Twenty-six patients met the eligibility criteria and were enrolled in the study. In one patient, it was not possible to visualize the ALL; in all other knees, where the ALL was identified, the ligament originated anterior and distal to the lateral epicondyle and was inserted on the proximal tibia approximately 5 mm below the joint line, just slightly posterior to Gerdy's tubercle (Fig. 8.11). The ALL had an average length of 33 ± 1.2 mm, an average width of 5.5 ± 0.3 mm, and an average thickness of 2 mm.

According to this study, the identification of the anterolateral ligament of the knee could sometimes be difficult due to adjacent structures, such as the anterolateral capsule, LCL (lateral collateral ligament), popliteus tendon, and iliotibial band (ITB), which cause a partial volume effect in the region and hamper the characterization of the ALL. However, a careful MRI evaluation was able to detect the ALL in 96% (25/26) of the patients.

A subsequent study evaluated MRI images of both knees in patients with acute ACL injuries, comparing the anatomy of the healthy side with the newly injured

Fig. 8.11 The anterolateral ligament is visible on 1.5 T2 magnetic resonance imaging scans in an uninjured knee. The arrow indicates the anterolateral ligament, and the arrowheads indicate the inferior lateral genicular vessels

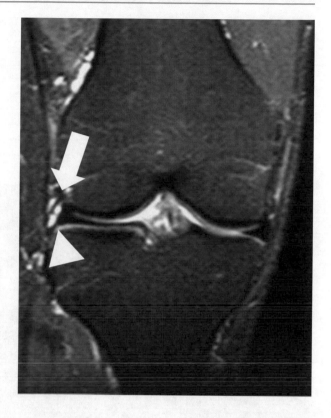

side [15]. A total of 36 patients were enrolled in the study. In two patients (5.5%), it was not possible to visualize the ALL in the uninjured knee, so these patients were excluded from the overall statistical analyses. Thus, 34 patients formed the final study population. Overall, 30 (88.2%) patients had at least one ALL abnormality in the ACL-injured knee. In 27 (79.4%) patients, the ALL showed an increased signal. In 22 (64.7%) knees, there were differences in the thickness of the ALL fibres, with an increased thickness in 15 (44.1%) knees and tapering in 7 (20.6%) knees. In 21 (61.7%) injured knees, irregularities were noted in the path of the ALL fibres. No cases of complete transection of the ALL or bony avulsion were found in this series. Asymmetry of the genicular vessels was observed in 21 (61.7%) injured knees (Table 8.1 and Figs. 8.12 and 8.13).

In summary, the most significant MRI changes observed in acute ACL tears included modifications of the ALL signal and thickness, an increase in the ALL signal and the disappearance of genicular vessels. These findings suggest that clinicians should have a high index of suspicion for ALL injuries when evaluating MRI scans of acutely ACL-injured knees, as changes can be identified in the majority of cases (approximately 90%) [15].

Table 8.1 Prevalence of anterolateral ligament abnormalities and associated lesions in knees with acute injury of the anterior cruciate ligament

Abnormality	N (%)
Any abnormality	30 (88.2%)
Signal change	27 (79.4%)
Thickness and thinness	22 (64.7%)
Fibre path	21 (61.7%)
Genicular vessel asymmetry	21 (61.7%)
Iliotibial bundle tear	12 (35.3%)

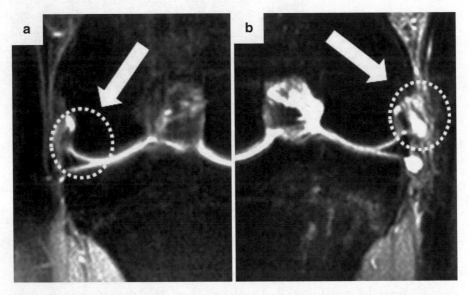

Fig. 8.12 Coronal T2-weighted magnetic resonance images (MRIs) with fat saturation of the (**a**) uninjured right knee and (**b**) injured left knee of a patient. The arrows and dotted circle indicate the anterolateral ligament. MRI of the left knee (**b**) demonstrated a slightly thickened anterolateral ligament with an increased signal compared with the contralateral side

Other studies reported a lower prevalence of all injuries associated with ACL tears. Van Dyck et al., in a series of patients examined within 8 weeks of their initial ACL injury, identified an ALL tear in 46% of the patients [16].

Won Lee et al., in a later study, documented a 64% prevalence of ALL tears in a series of 275 patients examined with MRI within five days after ACL injury [17].

In a further study, we compared MRI data with surgical findings to verify whether MRI could actually identify the pattern, site and severity of an anterolateral complex ligamentous injury.

The study [18] was based on a sample of 26 patients of acute anterolateral instability. Prior to the operation, the patients were examined by MRI and then operated on within 10 days of the trauma. The MRI scans were evaluated by three blinded observers. The fibres were considered abnormal when they presented irregular

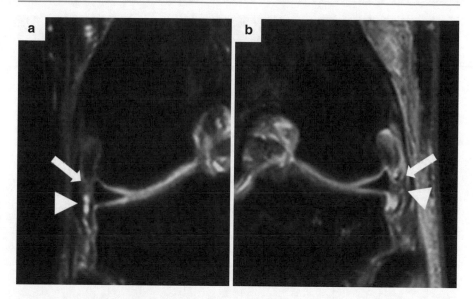

Fig. 8.13 Coronal T2-weighted magnetic resonance images with fat saturation of the (**a**) uninjured right knee and (**b**) injured left knee of a patient. The arrow indicates the anterolateral ligament, and the arrowheads indicate the inferior lateral genicular vessels. MRI of the left knee demonstrated a change in thickness and an increased signal of the anterolateral ligament compared with the contralateral normal ligament. The proximal fibres were also irregular. Note that the inferior lateral genicular vessels are asymmetric and are better depicted on the uninjured side (**a**)

contours, wavy aspects, or areas of discontinuity. Joint capsule lesions were defined by a thickening and increased signal in the T2-weighted sequences as well as the presence of periarticular fluid. The results showed that the ALL/anterolateral capsule was considered normal in 4 of the 26 (15.4%) patients and abnormal in 22 (84.6%) patients. Tears of the ALL and capsule were judged to be complete in 15 of the 22 (68.2%) patients and incomplete in seven (31.8%) patients.

At the time of surgery, the external compartment was explored, and possible injuries in that area were accurately described according to Ferretti et al.'s classification [19], recorded and eventually repaired. The ALL and capsule were found to be abnormal in 25 of the 26 patients (96.2%). The ALL and capsular tear were complete in 10 of the 25 (40.0%) patients and incomplete in 15 (60.0%) patients. The site of the capsular tear was limited to the anterior portion in 11 of the 25 (44.0%) patients and extended posteriorly in 14 (56.0%) patients.

In all cases, the fascia lata appeared to be substantially intact with no or minimal changes, possibly indicating only mildly stretching and/or haemorrhage. However, in the same cases, overflow was detected as soon as the subcutaneous tissue was released during surgery above the fascia lata; the presence of a thin layer of liquid, also detectable by careful examination of MRI imaging, indicated capsular damage and a possible increased permeability of the fascia (Fig. 8.14c).

The sensitivity, specificity, positive predictive value, negative predictive value, and accuracy of MRI for parameters of injury to the anterolateral structures of the

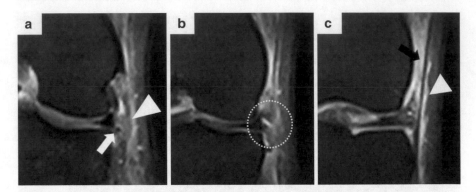

Fig. 8.14 Coronal T2-weighted magnetic resonance imaging of an acute tear in an injured left knee: (**a**) The arrowhead indicates the anterolateral ligament, and the arrow indicates one of the inferolateral genicular vessels. (**b**) The dotted circle indicates discontinuity of the ALL and lateral capsule which are surrounded by a thin layer of fluid below the subcutaneous region. (**c**) The black arrow indicates the iliotibial band with a normal signal and thickness; the white arrowhead indicates the presence of fluid localized between the subcutaneous tissue and fascia lata

Table 8.2 Correlation between MRI for parameters of injury to the anterolateral structures of the acute ACL-injured knee (based on surgical exploration as the gold standard)

	Sensitivity	Specificity	PPV	NPV	Accuracy
ITB Abnormality	62.5 (24.49–91.48)	40.0 (12.16–73.76)	45.5 (28.49–63.54)	57.1 (29.2–81.17)	50.0 (26.02–73.98)
ALL/capsule abnormality	88.0 (68.8–97.4)	100.0 (2.5–100.0)	100.0 (NA)	25.0 (10.34–49.07)	88.5 (69.85–97.55)
ALL/capsule complete/partial tear	78.6 (49.2–95.34)	41.7 (15.17–72.33)	61.1 (47.53–73.16)	62.5 (33.29–84.77)	61.5 (40.57–79.77)
ALL /capsule anterior/posterior	75.0 (34.91–98.61)	64.3 (35.14–87.24)	54.6 (34.83–72.93)	81.8 (56.02–94.08)	68.2 (45.13–86.14)

Values are presented as percentages (95% CI). Legend: *ACL* anterior cruciate ligament, *ALL* anterolateral ligament, *ITB* iliotibial band, *MRI* magnetic resonance imaging, *NA* not applicable, *NPV* negative predictive value, *PPV* positive predictive value

acute ACL-injured knee are reported in Table 8.2, with surgical exploration as the gold standard. The K test for the correlation between surgical and MRI findings is reported in Table 8.3, with the strength of agreement according to Altman.

Figures 8.14, 8.15, 8.16, 8.17 and 8.18 compare the MRI findings with the surgical findings.

In summary, on the basis of our experience with the use of MRI as a tool to pre-operatively detect ACL changes, especially in cases of acute injuries, we can postulate that MRI shows high sensitivity and specificity in identifying anterolateral capsular complex injuries. Therefore, surgeons can be confident in exploring the external compartment on the basis of MRI, with a good chance of finding anatomically and surgically relevant injuries of the ALL and capsule.

Table 8.3 Correlation between MRI and surgical findings: Cohen Kappa, Altman classification of strength of agreement and overall percentage agreement

	Kappa	Altman classification	Agreement %
ITB abnormality	0.27	Fair	65
ALL/capsule			
• Any abnormality	0.47	Moderate	88
• Determination of complete/partial tear	0.23	Fair	61
• Determination of anterior/posterior tear extension	0.49	Moderate	57

ALL anterolateral ligament, *ITB* iliotibial band, *MRI* magnetic resonance imaging

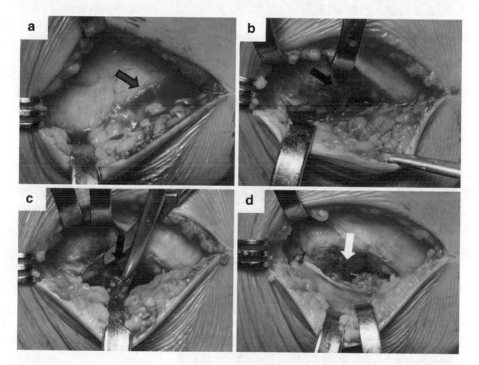

Fig. 8.15 Same case of Fig. 8.14. Surgical exploration. (**a**) Haemorrhagic fluid (red arrow) over an apparently normal fascia lata. (**b, c**) under the fascia lata, the capsule shows a complete tear of the anterolateral capsule and ligament (black arrows). (**d**) The white arrows indicate repair of the ALL and capsule

However, to date, protocols seem unable to more precisely detect the type and severity of an injury, even when a simplified classification (complete/incomplete) is used.

Sometimes, MRI can take several days to be performed, possibly resulting in a delayed operation; post-traumatic stiffness can occur and soft tissue may become less suitable for surgical repair, possibly increasing the risk of complications (arthrofibrosis).

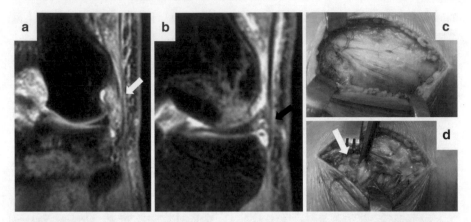

Fig. 8.16 Coronal T2-weighted magnetic resonance imaging: (**a**) Increased thickness of the proximal portion of the anterolateral ligament (white arrow) with marked regional oedema; (**b**) Decreased signal of the preinsertional iliotibial band (black arrow) characterized by adjacent oedema, with no fibre discontinuity. Surgical findings: (**c**) The fascia lata appeared moderately stretched and haemorrhagic with an incomplete preinsertional tear of fascia lata; (**d**) The capsule showing a complete tear of the anterolateral capsule and ligament (arrow)

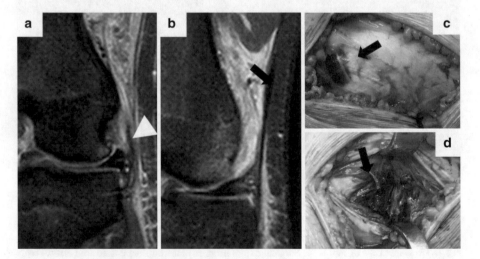

Fig. 8.17 Coronal T2-weighted magnetic resonance imaging showing incomplete ALL tears. (**a**) Anterolateral ligament (arrowheads) showing the uneven appearance of its fibres without signs of discontinuity; (**b**) Iliotibial band (black arrow) with a normal signal, thickness, and continuity. Surgical findings: (**c**) Stretching and haemorrhage on the distal fascia lata (black arrow) and (**d**) severe stretching and haemorrhage extending from the anterolateral ligament and capsule to the posterolateral capsule (black arrow). In this case, MRI underestimated the extent of the damage to the anterolateral complex

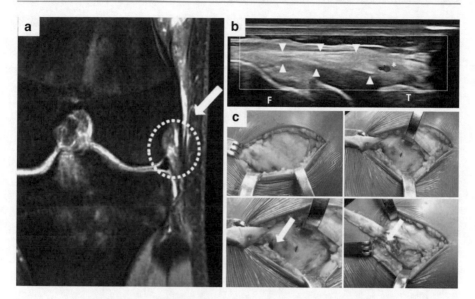

Fig. 8.18 (a) Coronal T2-weighted magnetic resonance images (MRIs) with fat saturation of the left injured knee: the dotted circle indicates that the anterolateral ligament presents an abnormal signal and irregular aspect of its fibres. ITB strain (arrow) with no fibre discontinuity. (b) US longitudinal image showing the thickness of the distal fibres of the ALL (arrowheads) with the inferolateral genicular vessels. (c) Surgical exploration of the normal fascia lata showing localized oedema without tears and more deeply showing the stretched anterolateral capsule

Therefore, as a reliable clinical diagnosis can be obtained in most cases, the actual need and advantages of MRI should be carefully assessed in each case.

In chronic cases, the chance to carry out a complete and reliable objective examination usually enables a reliable complete diagnosis, leading to an easy plan for the required treatment (conservative, isolated ACL reconstruction, combined intraarticular and extraarticular reconstruction).

However, as MRI is broadly used before surgery for chronic instabilities, we are getting used to carefully observing the external compartment, even in chronic cases. There is no doubt that in chronic cases, changes in the anterolateral complex are less visible, and often, these structures might appear perfectly normal.

Recovery of an apparently normal signal several weeks after injury has raised the question of the potential spontaneous healing of ALL injuries. This is an ongoing issue, and it is not easy to solve. There is no doubt that the ligaments of the external compartment, like all human ligaments, have a certain potential for self-healing to some extent, as all collagen healing processes are quite similar regardless of the type of ligament. However, even when the MRI signal is apparently normal, the actual tension and strength of the repaired tissue is impossible to assess. Therefore, in cases where the repaired ligament would be unable to recover adequate tension and strength, instability can occur even when an apparently normal signal is provided by MRI. To date, there are no reliable data to actually detect, based only on imaging data, the function of a repaired or healed ligament. Therefore, only biomechanics can provide reliable, even if indirect, proof of the actual function of a ligament.

In the literature, it is widely accepted that the level of pivot shift, in the case of an ACL-deficient knee, is related to injuries of secondary restraints. If anterolateral complex injuries heal with functionally acceptable scar tissue, even a few months after combined acute injury of the ACL and ALL, the phenomenon of pivot shifts should be reduced accordingly. However, in current clinical practice, this event is only seldom observed; in contrast, some months after injury, a worsening, rather than an improvement in rotational instability, is often detected. Therefore, we should assume that the spontaneous self-healing ability of anterolateral complex structures is limited.

In other words, the evidence of chronic instabilities with Pivot Shift +++ is all but rare, which proves a persistent insufficiency of both the ACL and its secondary restraints.

In conclusion, in chronic cases, the analyses of MRI concerning the anterolateral complex are less reliable, as the function of the ACL and other structures can mostly be assessed through an accurate objective examination and a correct evaluation and grading of the pivot shift test.

Furthermore, the presence of apparently normal structures, as detected by MRI, does not provide any reliable information about their biomechanics and function.

References

1. Geyer M, Wirth CJ. A new mechanism of injury of the anterior cruciate ligament. Unfallchirurg 1991.
2. Torg JS, Conrad W, Kalen V. Clinical diagnosis of anterior cruciate ligament instability in the athlete. Am J Sports Med. 1976;4:84.
3. Jakson LJ, O'Malley PJ, Kroenke K. Evaluation of acute knee pain in primary care. Ann Intern Med. 2003;139:575.
4. Mulligan PE, McGuffie DQ, Couner K, Khazzam M. The reliability and diagnostic accuracy of assessing the translation endpoint during the lachman test. Int J Sports Phys Ther. 2015;10:52.
5. Argento G, Vetrano M, Cristiano L, Suarez T, Bartoloni A, Erroi D, Ferretti A, Vulpiani MC. Ultrasonographic assessment of the anterolateral ligament of the knee in healthy subjects. Muscles Ligaments Tendons J. 2018;7:485.
6. Klos B, Scholtes M, Konijnenberg S. High prevalence of all complex Segond avulsion using ultrasound imaging. Knee Surg Sports Traumatol Arthrosc. 2017;25:1331.
7. Bock GW, Bosch E, Mishra DK, Daniel DM, Resnick D. The healed Segond fracture: a characteristic residual bone excrescence. Skeletal Radiol. 1994;23:555.
8. Campos JC, Chung CB, Lektrakul N, Pedowitz R, Trudell D, Yu J, Resnick D. Pathogenesis of the Segond fracture: anatomic and MR imaging evidence of an ileotibial tract avulsion. Radiology. 2001;
9. Claes S, Bartholomeeusen S, Bellemans J. High prevalence of anterolateral ligament abnormalities in magnetic resonance images of anterior cruciate ligament-injured knees. Acta Orthoped Belg. 2014;80:45.

10. Weber WN, Neumann CH, Barakos JA, Petersen SA, Steinbach LS, Genant HK. Lateral tibial rim (Segond) fractures: MR imaging characteristics. Radiology. 1991;180:731.
11. Hess T, Rupp S, Hopf T, Gleitz M, Liebler J. Lateral tibial avulsion fractures and disruptions to the anterior cruciate ligament: a clinical study of their incidence and correlation. Clin Orthop Relat Res. 1994;
12. Cavaignac E, Laumond G, Reina N, Wytrykowski K, Murgier J, Faruch M, Chiron P. How to test the anterolateral ligament with ultrasound. Arthrosc Tech. 2017;
13. Shekari I, Shekarchi B, Abbasian M, Sajjadi MM, Moghaddam AM, Kazemi SM. Predictive factors associated with anterolateral ligament injury in the patients with anterior cruciate ligament tear. Indian J Orthop. 2020;54:655.
14. De Carli A, Monaco E, Mazza D, Argento G, Redler A, Proietti L, et al. Assessment of the anterolateral ligament of the knee by magnetic resonance imaging. Joints. 2018;
15. Ferretti A, Monaco E, Redler A, Argento G, De Carli A, Saithna A, Partezani Helito PV, et al. High prevalence of anterolateral ligament abnormalities on MRI in knees with acute anterior cruciate ligament injuries: A case-control series from the SANTI study group. Orthop J Sports Med. 2019;7:6.
16. Van Dyck P, Clockaerts S, Vanhoenacker FM, Lambrecht V, Wouters K, De Smet E, et al. Anterolateral ligament abnormalities in patients with acute anterior cruciate ligament rupture are associated with lateral meniscal and osseous injuries. EurRadiol. 2016;26:3383.
17. Lee DW, Lee JH, Kim JN, Moon SG, Kim NR, Kim DH, et al. Evaluation of anterolateral ligament injuries and concomitant lesions on magnetic resonance imaging after acute anterior cruciate ligament rupture. Arthroscopy. 2018;34:2398.
18. Monaco E, Partezani Helito C, Redler A, Argento G, De Carli A, Saithna A, et al. Correlation between magnetic resonance imaging and surgical exploration of the anterolateral structures of the acute anterior cruciate ligament-injured knee. Am J Sports Med. 2019;47:1186.
19. Ferretti A, Monaco E, Fabbri M, Maestri M, De Carli A. Prevalence and classification of injuries of anterolateral complex in acute anterior cruciate ligament tears. Arthroscopy. 2016;

Why the Semitendinosus?

9

Andrea Ferretti, Luca Labianca, and Paola Papandrea

I clearly remember the first intra-articular ACL reconstruction performed in the historic building that housed the Orthopaedic Unit at the University La Sapienza Campus in Rome (Fig. 9.1).

It occurred in November 1979, and at that time, the most widespread and accredited techniques in Europe were those proposed by Kenneth Jones [1, 2], who used the patellar tendon, and by Lindemann [3], modified by Bousquet [4], who used the semitendinosus.

Giancarlo Puddu was the lead surgeon during this first historic surgery at our institute.

The chief of the department, Professor Lamberto Perugia, gave Giancarlo Puddu his full support simply because the original technique he developed used the semitendinosus graft as an ACL substitute.

As a young resident, I was allowed to attend this extraordinary event. It was the first of a long and successful series of ACL reconstructions.

During the following decades, Giancarlo Puddu and all members of our team grew in notoriety in the world of orthopaedics.

The reasons why Professor Perugia enthusiastically supported Giancarlo Puddu in the development of his ACL reconstruction technique were mainly biological and clinical.

From a biological point of view, Professor Perugia believed that the semitendinosus was more suitable for the synovial knee joint environment because, unlike the patellar tendon, it is surrounded by a thin and continuous synovial sheath.

A. Ferretti (✉)
Orthopaedic Unit, Sant'Andrea University Hospital, La Sapienza University, Rome, Italy

L. Labianca · P. Papandrea
Sant'Andrea Sapienza University Hospital, Rome, Italy

Fig. 9.1 The Orthopaedics
Department at the Campus
of the University La
Sapienza in Rome

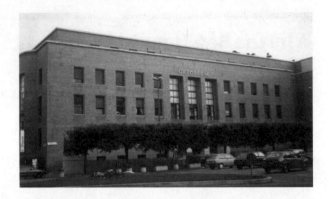

Clinically, the choice of the hamstring was suggested to avoid any possible weakening of the extensor knee mechanism resulting from the harvesting one-third of the patellar tendon with two bone plugs from the patella and the tibia site.

At that time, in the 1970s, the first studies on patellar tendon pain were presented, and patellar tendinopathy was recognized and clearly defined as a distinct clinical entity [5–8].

All the surgeons on our team were perfectly aware of the potential risk that harvesting one-third of the patellar tendon may have on the biomechanics and function of the extensor mechanism, which could possibly lead to anterior knee pain, patella baja, patellar tendinopathy and other issues.

On the other hand, harvesting hamstrings seemed to be less invasive and less risky for knee biomechanics.

However, in the 1990s, mainly because in the USA many surgeons strongly supported using the bone-patellar tendon-bone (BPTB) (as a free graft and no longer attached to the tibial tuberosity), the BPTB became the global gold standard in the treatment of ACL-deficient knees.

Nevertheless, in the La Sapienza University Orthopaedic Unit, the hamstrings remained the graft of choice. The results we recorded, compared to those reported in the literature using patellar tendon graft for ACL reconstruction techniques, eventually showed a lower rate of complications due to the lower donor site morbidity of the technique.

Moreover, intra-articular reconstruction with hamstrings was often associated with extra-articular reconstruction in selected cases.

The strength of the semitendinosus and gracilis graft, compared to the native ACL and patellar tendon, was another matter of debate.

The biomechanical properties of a graft are a crucial issue in the selection of the ACL substitute. Therefore, several studies have investigated the mechanical properties of either the semitendinosus and gracilis graft or the patellar tendon graft.

Hamner and Brown are mainly credited for having shown that the main mechanical prerequisite of a quadrupled, equal tensioned hamstring graft, including the strength and stiffness, is statistically higher than those of the central third of the patellar tendon and of the native ACL itself [9].

These findings supported the hypothesis that the hamstring graft could be a suitable biomechanical choice for ACL reconstruction [10].

Another crucial difference between hamstring and BPTB grafts is the two bone plugs at the extremities of the patellar tendon, feasibly resulting in a stronger initial fixation, in addition to faster and better integration and biological, definitive, fixation and integration of the graft inside the bone tunnels (bone to bone for the patellar tendon, tendon to bone for hamstrings).

All hamstring users were well aware of the lower mechanical strength of tendon-to-bone (TTB) fixation compared to bone-to-bone (BTB), whether the same devices were used (interference screws).

At that point, the issue became to develop a dedicated fixation device for allowing a stronger and more reliable mechanical fixation of a hamstring graft inside the bone tunnel. We started studying and developing new and reliable fixation devices that could be able to gain the same mechanical results as BTB fixation, eventually promoting faster and safer biological integration of the graft.

The aim of our research was to develop fixation devices specific for the use of hamstrings with higher mechanical properties, such as strength and stiffness, to ensure safe initial fixation of the graft, avoiding any disturbance to definitive biological fixation.

The first device developed by our group was that of the femoral side, where the loop of the doubled tendons offers a better and easier attachment point.

Once the femoral fixation device was studied and set, we faced the more challenging issue of fixation on the tibial side.

The two main problems on this side are the lower resistance to slippage of the free ends of the tendons and the reduced bone density of the proximal tibia compared with the distal femur. Even the use of two staples in a belt buckle fashion was somehow biomechanically disappointing.

The first device developed in our department was the Swing Bridge (Citieffe, Bologna, Italy) [11] (Fig. 9.2), a patented cortical suspension device for the femoral

Fig. 9.2 The Swing Bridge device

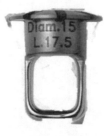

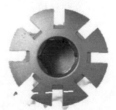

fixation of looped tendons, designed for use in cases of outside-in femoral drilling only.

The device is composed of a titanium-alloy cylinder (diameter, 10 mm) with a smooth metal half-ring (diameter, 10 mm) on one end and a shelf with grooves on the other. When performing an outside-in technique, the free tendon ends are threaded through the device's ring and then pulled into the joint. The cylinder is inserted into the femoral tunnel with an impactor until the shelf reaches the femoral cortical bone. If the surgeon judges that the tension of the graft is not satisfactory after tibial fixation, the Swing Bridge allows further tensioning of the graft by rotating the device that twists the graft bundles [12].

The main and unique characteristic of the Swing Bridge was that it allowed the surgeon to tune the tension of the graft (according to the surgeon's judgement) once the graft was fixed at the tibial side by simply rotating the device up to 360 degrees or more (Fig. 9.3). In this way, twisting the graft bundle is able to improve graft tension.

The ultimate tension of the graft could be easily assessed arthroscopically. This procedure aims to reduce the risk of any loss of graft tension possibly occurring after tibial fixation.

Fig. 9.3 The Swing Bridge tensioning system as first used along with two staples in a belt buckle fashion for tibial fixation (reprinted with permission from Citieffe catalogue, Bologna, Italy)

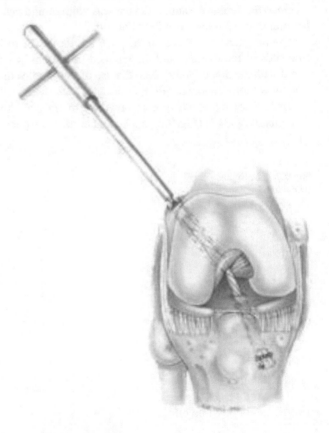

Table 9.1 Mean Stiffness and Pull-out strength of the Swing Bridge (Citieffe, Bologna, Italy) as compared with the most popular femoral fixation device of the late nineties (Endobutton Continuous Loop, Smith and Nephew, Andover, MA, USA)

	Stiffness	Pull-out strength
Swing Bridge	218 N/mm	1181 N
Endobutton/continuous loop	118 N/mm	1226 N
Statistical significance ($\alpha<0.05$)	$\alpha<0.05$	$\alpha>0.05$

Moreover, because of the well-known viscoelasticity of the tendons, progressive elongation of the graft possibly occurs after the procedure, with a partial loss of the stability obtained at surgery due to progressive stretching of the graft.

For this reason, adequate pretensioning and proper tensioning of the graft during fixation would avoid this issue, eventually increasing knee stability at follow-up.

The Swing Bridge was tested in one of the most equipped laboratories, the biomechanical laboratory of the Women's and Brigham Hospital at Harvard University in Boston, by some of the most experts in this specific field [13].

Biomechanical properties such as strength and stiffness were evaluated and compared with the most popular and reliable suspension device, the Endobutton continuous loop (Smith and Nephew, Andover, Ma), in a series of cadaver knees.

As shown in Table 9.1, the Swing Bridge values were comparable to the Endobutton CL values in the pull-out strength test, while the stiffness was significantly higher than that provided by the Endobutton CL.

Once the Swing Bridge obtained definitive approval by health authorities, our research switched towards the more challenging tibial fixation.

After a series of studies and laboratory tests, a new device was eventually developed, approved and became commercially available: the Evolgate (Citieffe, Bologna, Italy) [14].

The Evolgate is composed of three items made with titanium alloy: a spiral, screw and washer.

After the tunnel is properly drilled, a spiral (2 cm long, 1 mm thick) is inserted into the distal half of the tibial tunnel with a dedicated impactor. The goal of this spiral is to strengthen the bone walls of the tunnel. Once the free ends of the hamstring graft are pulled down from the distal end of the tunnel, a screw is screwed in deeply, squeezing the tendons towards the coil of the spiral and bone walls, providing secure fixation of the graft. Last, a washer provides a cortical grip, pushing the tendons down at the exit of the bone tunnel.

The result is a combination of internal interference fixation and external cortical compression (Fig. 9.4).

Several laboratory studies have evaluated the mechanical properties of the Evolgate as well as those of the Swing-Bridge-Tendons-Evolgate complex compared with other coupled popular fixation devices (Figs. 9.5 and 9.6) [15, 16].

Moreover, the Evolgate has also been studied from a biological point of view to investigate its possible effect on the definitive biological fixation of the graft. The

Fig. 9.4 The Evolgate
fixation system (reprinted
with permission from
Citieffe catalogue,
Bologna, Italy)

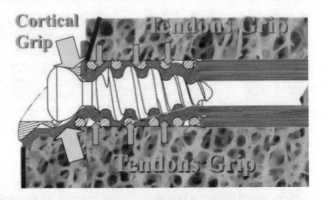

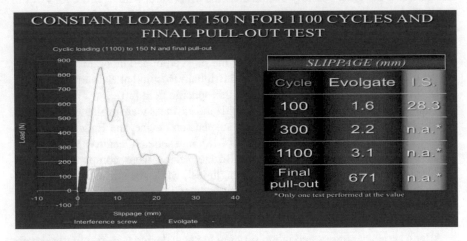

Fig. 9.5 Pull-out test after 1100 cycles at a constant load of 150 N. Note the greater slippage and lower strength of the interference screw compared with the Evolgate. Green: Interference screw; Red: Evolgate

bone–tendon interface was histologically evaluated in vivo in sheep, in which an Evolgate was implanted in the tibias to securely fix a tendon into a bone tunnel.

The bone–tendon junction was histologically evaluated at 4 and 12 weeks after surgery and revealed the presence of secure biological direct fixations through well-visible Sharpey fibres (Fig. 9.7) [17]

We can now reasonably state that the Evolgate, which we have used with excellent clinical results and no interruption since 2001, is one of the most studied and reliable tibial fixation devices, providing excellent fixation of the free ends of a graft.

Currently, even if the Evolgate is still successfully used in primary ACL reconstruction, its main indication relies on revision cases when a hamstring graft is used, and the bone density of the proximal tibia is supposed to be even weaker as a result of previous tunnelling or bone loss eventually resulting from the removal of previous fixation devices [18, 19].

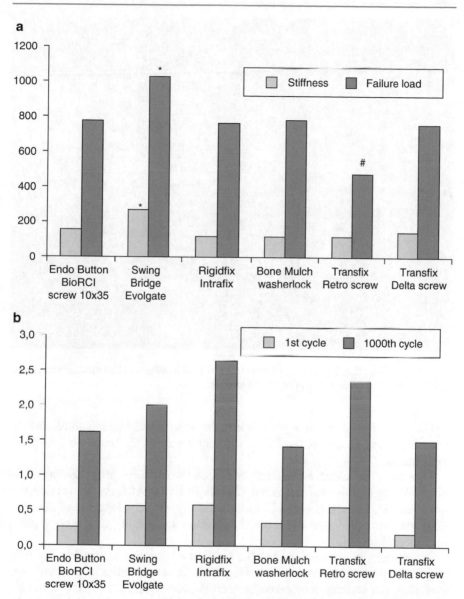

Fig. 9.6 (**a**) Pull-out strength (Newton) and (**b**) cyclic loading mechanical test (mm of slippage at the 1st and 1000th cycle) comparing several coupled femur and tibial fixation devices in a porcine model

However, a possible gap could still persist between the two techniques (BPTB and hamstrings) in terms of the biological fixation timing provided by bone-to-bone healing, which is supposed to occur much faster than tendon-to-bone healing.

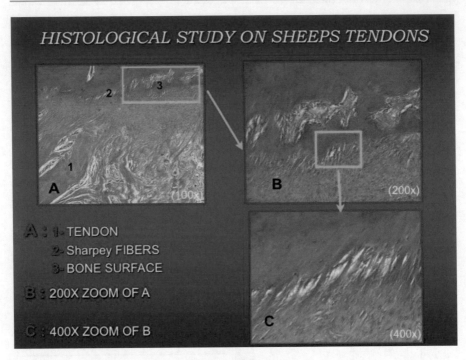

Fig. 9.7 Histology showing Sharpey fibres at bone–tendon interface at 12 weeks (biological fixation as provided by the Evolgate in an animal model)

The actual fate of the bone plugs inside the bone tunnel was unknown, and the better biological healing of the BPTB technique was mainly based on theoretical speculations.

Therefore, to better understand the process of bone plug healing once recessed into the femoral and tibial tunnels in BPTB ACL reconstruction, we performed a CT study of knees 12 months postoperatively. Imaging of the bone plugs was examined, and the actual integration and vitality of the bone plugs were evaluated [20].

Surprisingly, in only one-third of the cases, the bone plug was viable and fully integrated into the surrounding bone (Fig. 9.8). In another third of the cases, the bone plug was partially reabsorbed or necrotic, and in the last third, it was fully reabsorbed and no longer identifiable by CT (Fig. 9.9).

Therefore, based on the results of this study, the ability of a BPTB graft to provide fast and secure biological fixation in most cases should be strongly questioned, with definitive fixation, in at least one-third of cases, provided by a tendon-to-bone healing; likewise, this also happens with hamstring grafts.

Fig. 9.8 CT scan 13 months after ACL reconstruction with a BPTB graft showing complete osteointegration of the bone plug. This favourable outcome occurs in no more than one-third of cases

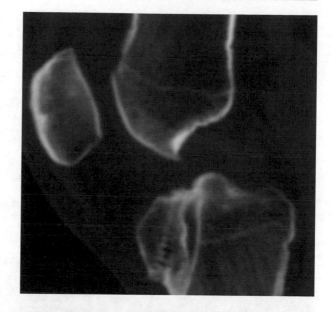

Fig. 9.9 CT scan 12 months after ACL reconstruction with BPTB showing complete resorption of the bone plug in the tibial tunnel

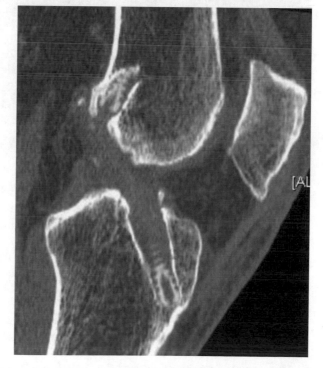

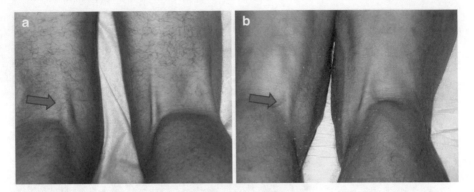

Fig. 9.10 Clinical evaluation at 4 months (**a**) postop. The ticker regenerated semitendinosus tendon is outlined by the arrow. At 1 year (**b**) postop, the ST tendon appears to be almost indistinguishable from a normal one

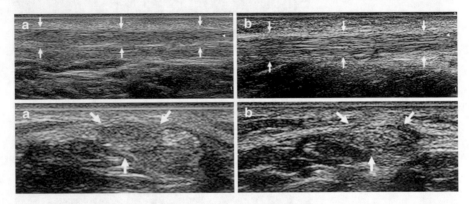

Fig. 9.11 (**a, b**) Longitudinal fibres and transverse fibres echoscan at 10 months comparing [**a**] affected and [**b**] normal side

Another crucial factor we have carefully investigated is the fate of the flexor mechanism and semitendinosus tendon once fully harvested for reconstruction.

Initially, possible regeneration of the tendon was visible as an appreciable, larger than normal, string in the medial edge of the popliteal fossa a few weeks postoperatively. The tension was significantly increased during active flexion of the knee; since 12 months after surgery, a quite normal regenerated semitendinosus could be clinically observed, essentially indistinguishable from the contralateral semitendinosus (Fig. 9.10a, b).

Then, a sequential ultrasound study was performed (at 2 weeks and 1, 2, 3, 6, 12, 18, and 24 months postoperatively) to evaluate the anatomy and structure of the regenerated tissue [21].

The results of this study showed the early formation of longitudinally oriented scar tissue that progressively developed the shape, structure and echogenicity of the native (contralateral) semitendinosus within a few months (Fig. 9.11).

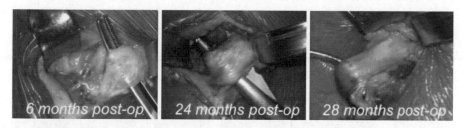

Fig. 9.12 Intraoperative findings of the regenerated semitendinosus during second surgeries in three different patients

At 18 months postoperatively, the regenerated semitendinosus appeared to be essentially indistinguishable from a normal semitendinosus.

Later, we had the chance to directly inspect the regenerated tendon during second surgeries to remove painful or disturbing tibial fixation devices (staples) (Fig. 9.12) [22].

Several biopsies were taken, and the harvested tissue was examined histologically. In all samples, a longitudinally well-arranged array of fibres was found with a large count of cells resembling young tenocytes.

However, clinical features, as well as US imaging, later supported by MRI, revealed that the regenerated semitendinosus eventually inserted over the popliteal fascia rather than on the pes anserinus, possibly resulting in a loss of any internal rotation strength of the muscle.

To preserve internal rotation, a modified harvesting technique was proposed [23]. Taking advantage of the length of the tendons, which normally exceeded the required length for ACL reconstruction, we saved the distal end of the tendons from the insertion to 3 cm.

This would produce a kind of scaffold for the new tendon, possibly recovering its original pathway towards the pes anserinus.

In our experience, this modified harvesting technique actually resulted in a restored, stronger internal rotation of the hamstrings.

However, despite the possible partial loss of strength due to muscle retraction of the semitendinosus (well documented by MRI studies, the Starling law), with proper rehabilitation, the difference with the unaffected site could be reduced (Fig. 9.13).

Since the beginning of this century, when many surgeons worldwide reconsidered the hamstrings as a valid alternative to BPTB grafts, many clinical studies have been published comparing the two techniques. Today, there is a general agreement that few differences actually exist in terms of restoring function and postoperative knee stability [24–26].

However, a lower rate of failure and the recurrence of instability have been reported when a BPTB graft is used. This issue still leads to the consideration of a BPTB graft as a preferred choice in the case of high-level athletes involved in high-risk sports.

In our experience with professional football players who underwent ACL reconstruction with BPTB grafts and returned to the preoperative level of activity, despite

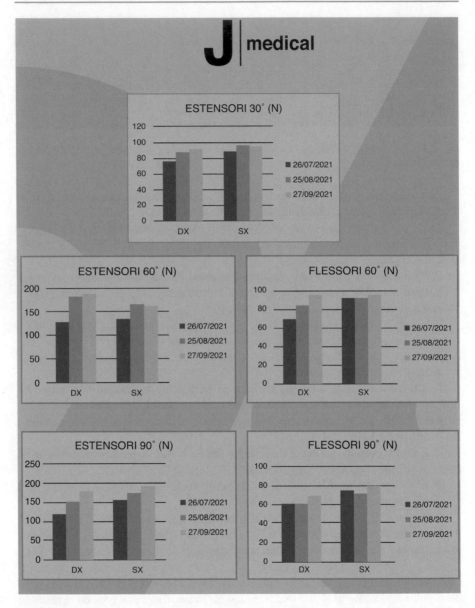

Fig. 9.13 ACL reconstruction with the hamstrings and extra-articular reconstruction in the right knee in a professional football player (a woman). A muscle evaluation four months after proper rehabilitation was performed. Both the extensor and flexor muscular strength appeared to be almost completely restored. Dx: right. Sx: left (courtesy of J Medical Lab, Torino, Italy)

very good knee stability, a mild loss of extension was often observed, as revealed by examining the height of the heels in the prone position.

This condition could be defined as mild stiffness that could contribute to the feeling of stability perceived by the examiner and referenced by the patient.

To our knowledge, very few studies have compared the clinical results of ACL reconstruction with BPTB grafts with hamstrings when extra-articular reconstruction (EAR) is added.

Zaffagnini et al. [27] and, more recently, Rota et al. [28] evaluated three cohorts of patients who underwent BPTB grafts, hamstring grafts and hamstring grafts plus extra-articular reconstruction. Both studies documented that the best results were observed in the group of patients who underwent combined intra-articular reconstruction with hamstrings and EAR.

Another very important concern in comparing BPTB and hamstring grafts is the influence of each procedure in promoting degenerative osteoarthrosis (DOA), as highlighted by the early appearance of its typical radiological changes.

Our experience in long-term follow-up studies strongly agrees with the recent literature, which accredited hamstring ACL reconstruction with a lower rate of radiological signs of DOA at medium-and long-term follow-ups [29–31].

The even mild change in knee mechanics resulting from the loss of the last few degrees of extension, often observed as a result of ACL reconstruction with BPTB graft, could reasonably explain this issue.

In conclusion, the use of semitendinosus and gracilis as grafts of choice in ACL reconstruction is supported by the following considerations:

Biological:

(a) The presence of a synovial sheath surrounding the semitendinosus and gracilis could reasonably promote the suitability of the graft to the articular environment.
(b) Reliable bone-to-tendon healing through Sharpey fibres (indirect fixation).
(c) The excellent potential for regeneration of the semitendinosus tendon.

Biomechanical:

(a) The excellent strength and stiffness to either cyclic loads or pull-out tests of a quadrupled, equally tensioned hamstring graft
(b) The possible use of fixation devices with excellent mechanical properties, also promoting biological fixation

Clinical:

(a) Low morbidity of the harvest site
(b) Very good short-term and long-term clinical results in terms of knee stability, recovery of function and return to sport, which could be strongly and easily implemented by the use of extra-articular reconstruction as an adjunct in selected cases and risky patients
(c) Lower risk of development of post-traumatic DOA

References

1. Jones KG. Reconstruction of the anterior cruciate ligament using the central one-third of the patellar ligament. J Bone Joint Surg Am. 1970;52(4):838–9.
2. Jones KG. Reconstruction of the anterior cruciate ligament. A technique using the central one-third of the patellar ligament. J Bone Joint Surg Am. 1963;45:925–32.
3. Lindemann K. Plastic surgery in substitution of the cruciate ligaments of the knee-joint by means of pedunculated tendon transplants. Zeitschrift für Orthopädie und ihre Grenzgebiete. 1950;79(2):316–34.
4. Bousquet G. Les indications thérapeutiques dans les laxités chroniques du genou. 5ème journées lyonnaises de chirurgie du genou. 1984; P 211–18.
5. Ferretti A, Ippolito E, Mariani P, Puddu G. Jumper's knee. Am J Sports Med. 1983;11(2):58–62. https://doi.org/10.1177/036354658301100202.
6. Ferretti A, Puddu G, Mariani PP, Neri M. The natural history of jumper's knee. Patellar or quadriceps tendonitis. Int Orthop. 1985;8(4):239–42. https://doi.org/10.1007/BF00266866.
7. Ferretti A. Epidemiology of jumper's knee. Sports Med. 1986;3(4):289–95. https://doi.org/10.2165/00007256-198603040-00005.
8. Mariani PP, Puddu G, Ferretti A. Jumper's knee. Ital J Orthop Traumatol. 1978;4(1):85–93.
9. Hamner DL, Brown CH Jr, Steiner ME, et al. Hamstring tendon grafts for reconstruction of the anterior cruciate ligament: biomechanical evaluation of the use of multiple strands and tensioning techniques. J Bone Joint Surg [Am]. 1999;81:549–57.
10. Brown CH Jr, Steiner ME, Carson EW. The use of hamstring tendons for anterior cruciate ligament reconstruction. Clin Sports Med. 1993;12:723–56.
11. Ferretti A, Conteduca F. Ricostruzione del legamento crociato anteriore coi tendini del semitendinoso e gracile raddoppiati: tecnica originale di tensionamento, fissazione ed avvolgimento dei fasci "Swing Bridge" (Ponte girevole). Italian J Orthop Traumatol. 1997;23:433–41.
12. Ferretti A, Conteduca F, Morelli F, Monteleone L, Nanni F, Valente M. Biomechanics of anterior cruciate ligament reconstruction using twisted doubled hamstring tendons. Int Orthop. 2003;27(1):22–5. https://doi.org/10.1007/s00264-002-0395-8. Epub 2002 Aug 13. PMID: 12582804; PMCID: PMC3673694
13. Brown CH, Ferretti A, Conteduca F, Morelli F, Hecker Wilson D. Biomechanics of the Swing-Bridge technique for anterior cruciate ligament reconstruction. Eur J Sports Traumatol Relat Res. 2001;23(2):69–73.
14. Ferretti A, Conteduca F, Morelli F, Ticca L, Monaco E. The Evolgate: a method to improve the pullout strength of interference screws in tibial fixation of ACL reconstruction with doubled gracilis and semitendinosus tendons. Arthroscopy. 2003;9:936–40.
15. Labianca L, Monaco E, Speranza A, Camillieri G, Ferretti A. Biomechanical evaluation of six femurgraft-tibia complexes in ACL reconstruction. J Orthop Traumatol. 2006;7(3):131–5. https://doi.org/10.1007/s10195-006-0136-7.
16. Monaco E, Fabbri M, Lanzetti R, Del Duca A, Labianca L, Ferretti A. Biomechanical comparison of four coupled fixation systems for ACL reconstruction with bone socket or full-tunnel on the tibial side. Knee. 2017;24:795–10.
17. Ferretti A, Monaco E, Labianca L, D'Angelo F, De Carli A, Conteduca F. How four and twelve weeks of implantation affect the strength and stiffness of a tendon graft securely fixed in a bone tunnel: a study of Evolgate fixation in an extra-articular model ovine model. J Orthop Traumatol. 2006;7(3):136–41. https://doi.org/10.1007/s10195-006-0138-5.
18. Ferretti A, Conteduca F, Monaco E, De Carli A, D'Arrigo C. Revision anterior cruciate ligament reconstruction with doubled semitendinosus and gracilis tendons and lateral extra-articular reconstruction. J Bone Joint Surg Am. 2006;88(11):2373–9. https://doi.org/10.2106/JBJS.F.00064.
19. Iorio R, Vadalà A, Argento G, Di Sanzo V, Ferretti A. Bone tunnel enlargement after ACL reconstruction using autologous hamstring tendons: a CT study. Int Orthop. 2007;31(1):49–55. https://doi.org/10.1007/s00264-006-0118-7. Epub 2006 May 9. PMID: 16683112

20. Vadalà A, Iorio R, Redler A, Valeo L, Ferretti M, Camillieri G, Argento G, Conteduca F, Ferretti A. Biological fixation of the bone graft in anterior cruciate ligament reconstruction with bone-patellar tendon-bone: does the bone plug really heal inside the tibial tunnel? A ct study. Poster Presentation at the American Academy of Orthopaedic Surgeons 2011 Annual Meeting at the San Diego Convention Center from February 15–19, 2011.
21. Papandrea P, Vulpiani MC, Ferretti A, Conteduca F. Regeneration of the semitendinosus tendon harvested for anterior cruciate ligament reconstruction. Evaluation using ultrasonography. Am J Sports Med. 2000;28(4):556–61. https://doi.org/10.1177/03635465000280041901.
22. Ferretti A, Conteduca F, Morelli F, Masi V. Regeneration of the semitendinosus tendon after its use in Anterior Cruciate Ligament: a histologic study of three cases. Am J Sports Med. 2002;30:204–7.
23. Ferretti A, Vadalà A, De Carli A, Argento G, Conteduca F, Severini G. Minimizing internal rotation strength deficit after use of semitendinosus for anterior cruciate ligament reconstruction: a modified harvesting technique. Arthroscopy. 2008;24(7):786–95. https://doi.org/10.1016/j.arthro.2008.02.010. Epub 2008 Apr 21
24. Mohtadi NG, Chan DS, Dainty KN, Whelan DB. Patellar tendon versus hamstring tendon autograft for anterior cruciate ligament rupture in adults. Cochrane Database Syst Rev. 2011;2011(9):CD005960.   https://doi.org/10.1002/14651858.CD005960.pub2.   PMID: 21901700; PMCID: PMC6465162
25. Mouarbes D, Menetrey J, Marot V, Courtot L, Berard E, Cavaignac E. Anterior cruciate ligament reconstruction: a systematic review and meta-analysis of outcomes for quadriceps tendon autograft versus bone-patellar tendon-bone and Hamstring-Tendon Autografts. Am J Sports Med. 2019;47(14):3531–40. https://doi.org/10.1177/0363546518825340. Epub 2019 Feb 21
26. Samuelsen BT, Webster KE, Johnson NR, Hewett TE, Krych AJ. Hamstring autograft versus patellar tendon autograft for acl reconstruction: is there a difference in graft failure rate? A meta-analysis of 47,613 patients. Clin Orthop Relat Res. 2017;475(10):2459–68. https://doi.org/10.1007/s11999-017-5278-9. PMID: 28205075; PMCID: PMC5599382
27. Zaffagnini S, Marcacci M, Lo Presti M, Giordano G, Iacono F, Neri MP. Prospective and randomized evaluation of ACL reconstruction with three techniques: a clinical and radiographic evaluation at 5 years follow-up. Knee Surg Sports Traumatol Arthrosc. 2006;14(11):1060–9. https://doi.org/10.1007/s00167-006-0130-x. Epub 2006 Aug 15
28. Rota P, Monaco E, Carrozzo A, Bruni G, Rota A, Ferretti A. Long-term clinical and radiographic results of ACL reconstruction: retrospective comparison between three techniques (Hamstrings Autograft, Hamstrings Autograft with Extra-Articular Reconstruction, Bone Patellar Tendon Autograft). Muscles Ligaments Tendons Journal. 2020;10(3):460–9. https://doi.org/10.32098/mltj.03.2020.15.
29. Freedman KB, D'Amato MJ, Nedeff DD, Kaz A, Bach BR Jr. Arthroscopic anterior cruciate ligament reconstruction: a metaanalysis comparing patellar tendon and hamstring tendon autografts. Am J Sports Med. 2003;31(1):2–11. https://doi.org/10.1177/03635465030310011501.
30. Ponzo A, Monaco E, Basiglini L, Iorio R, Caperna L, Drogo P, Conteduca F, Ferretti A. Long-term results of anterior cruciate ligament reconstruction using Hamstring Grafts and the outside-in technique: a comparison between 5- and 15-year follow-up. Orthop J Sports Med. 2018;6(8):2325967118792263. https://doi.org/10.1177/2325967118792263. PMID: 31457062; PMCID: PMC6700944
31. Xie X, Xiao Z, Li Q, Zhu B, Chen J, Chen H, Yang F, Chen Y, Lai Q, Liu X. Increased incidence of osteoarthritis of knee joint after ACL reconstruction with bone-patellar tendon-bone autografts than hamstring autografts: a meta-analysis of 1,443 patients at a minimum of 5 years. Eur J Orthop Surg Traumatol. 2015;25(1):149–59. https://doi.org/10.1007/s00590-014-1459-3. Epub 2014 Apr 21

Extra-Articular Reconstructions in ACL-Deficient Knee

10

Andrea Ferretti, Edoardo Monaco, and Alessandro Carrozzo

10.1 Background

Since the beginning of modern anterior cruciate ligament (ACL) surgery, when rotational instability and the pivot shift phenomenon were identified and described in ACL-deficient knees, extra-articular reconstructions (ERs) have been very popular. In 1968, Slocum and Larson stated that *"one of the most fascinating facets of the problem of knee ligament injuries is rotatory instability"* and focused on rotatory instability that occurred in ACL-deficient knees. The diagnostic value of the rotatory instability test was also emphasized [1].

Anterolateral rotatory instability (ALRI) can be easily demonstrated by the pivot shift test, which was described in 1972 [2]. The pivot shift test consists of a sudden rotation of the tibia relative to the femur for an ACL-injured knee under valgus torque at low angles of knee flexion. This comprises two components:

The rotational component: the internal rotation of the tibia about its long axis.
The translational component: anterior subluxation of the lateral tibial plateau followed by its sudden reduction under certain loading conditions [3].

At that time, well before arthroscopy and arthroscopic-related techniques had spread, some surgeons had already proposed the treatment of rotational instability by performing only ERs, and several techniques were described by many pioneer knee surgeons in the seventies and eighties, such as Hughston, Andrews, Ellison, and McIntosh et al. [4].

A. Ferretti (✉) · E. Monaco · A. Carrozzo
Orthopaedic Unit, Sant'Andrea University Hospital, La Sapienza University, Rome, Italy

© The Author(s), under exclusive license to Springer Nature Switzerland AG 2022
A. Ferretti (ed.), *Anterolateral Rotatory Instability in ACL Deficient Knee*,
https://doi.org/10.1007/978-3-031-00115-4_10

These techniques were mainly based on rotational control of the tibia by performing lateral tenodesis, similar to the first technique described by Lemaire in France. Currently, Lemaire's technique is recognized as the first and most popular technique for ERs, and it is still used worldwide, with some recent modifications [5]. Moreover, at that time, ACL reconstruction was performed by open surgery, and accurate anatomical placement of the graft was very difficult.

ERs, either isolated or in association with rough, very invasive, open, and poorly anatomical intraarticular ACL reconstructions, have remained popular since the eighties, when a consensus conference on this topic was organized by the AOSSM in Snowmass, Colorado.

Snowmass is a tiny village in the mountains of Colorado, but it has an important place in the history of orthopaedics, having hosted the consensus conference in 1989. This specific conference focused on the role of ERs in the surgical treatment of ACL-deficient knees. A panel of experts selected among the most renowned knee surgeons of that time, including J. Andrews, J. Bergfeld, W. Clancy, J. Feagin, R. Larson, F. Noyes, L. Paulos, B. Reider, and R. Steadman, gathered to discuss and share their experiences with ERs.

Five study groups were formed to have in-depth discussions on the following topics:

- The biomechanics of extra-articular reconstructions
- Extra-articular reconstruction in a skeletally immature knee
- Extra-articular reconstruction as the primary procedure in ACL-deficient knees
- Extra-articular reconstruction as a secondary support procedure in conjunction with intraarticular reconstruction in acute anterior cruciate-deficient knees
- Extra-articular reconstruction as a secondary support procedure in conjunction with intraarticular reconstruction in chronic anterior cruciate-deficient knees

As a result of the publication of the proceedings of this conference—collected by Arthur Pearle and John Bergfeld and published in a booklet by Human Kinetics in 1992 (Fig. 10.1)—ERs were almost completely abandoned in the USA. Indeed, according to Pearl and Bergfeld, Snowmass experts concluded that ERs were unable to provide any substantial advantage over isolated intraarticular reconstructions (IRs) and that they eventually resulted in increased morbidity, a higher risk of complications, and late osteoarthritis (OA). This booklet became the cornerstone of a new era of ACL reconstructions, aimed exclusively at replacing torn ACLs. Since then, the goal of most surgeons has been to accurately replicate the native ACL by precise identification of the ligament anatomy, including bundles and footprints. Taking advantage of the evolution of arthroscopic techniques and dedicated instruments, this approach runs together with the desire to ultimately reduce the morbidity of the procedure. The message was clear: isolated, properly executed ACL reconstruction is the best way to treat ACL-deficient knees, resulting in negative Lachman and pivot shift tests. All other ligamentous structures as well as any other surgical steps are of little, if any, value [6].

Fig. 10.1 The cover of the booklet where the proceedings of the Snowmass meeting were held

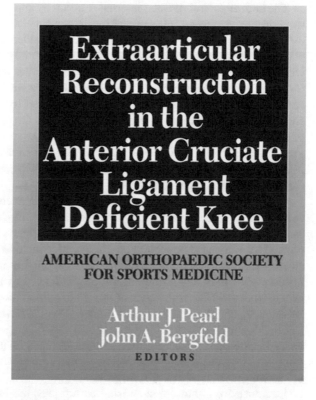

Moreover, arthroscopy itself led the surgeons to focus their attention only on tears of intraarticular structures, in fact disregarding all extra-articular structures that are not visible with a scope. As a result, injuries of anterolateral structures, well described decades earlier as secondary restraint of the ACL and an essential compo- nent of anterolateral rotatory instability, were no longer considered. Only a few years later, a minimally invasive procedure represented by a single incision bone- patellar tendon-bone (BPTB) nonanatomic transtibial reconstruction became the gold standard of ACL reconstructions [7].

However, some surgeons in a few centres around the world did not abandon the pathway traced by old textbooks of knee surgery and continued to perform strictly anatomic ACL reconstruction. Taking advantage of arthroscopy, they attempted to respect the native ACL anatomy even more thoroughly, using the hamstrings as a graft of choice and the two-incision technique to independently drill the femoral tunnel outside-in. They also continued to treat associated extra-articular lesions to address anterolateral rotational instability more comprehensively in ACL- deficient knees.

However, after almost two decades, many authors have reported a failure rate of 20% of more after isolated ACL reconstruction, with an unacceptable postoperative persistence of rotational instability and the pivot shift phenomenon [8].

The lack of control of tibial internal rotation by capsular anterolateral structures was considered as a possible cause of this unacceptable rate of failure [9]. Therefore, in the last decade, ERs have been strongly reconsidered, especially thanks to the obstinacy of some researchers from prestigious schools of orthopaedics in Europe, whose anatomical, biomechanical, and clinical studies represent a true benchmark for many knee surgeons around the world. Orthopaedic surgeons from France, the Netherlands, and of course Italy should be credited for their continuous, faithful, and effective contributions to the understanding of the role of ERs in the treatment of ACL-deficient knees. *However, why can ERs be reconsidered after a detailed report such as that coming from the Snowmass conference?* In fact, several changes have occurred in ACL surgery since the early 1980s, and the approach to ACL reconstruction has changed radically.

In fact, the experts at the time of the Snowmass meeting were extremely concerned about possible complications related to any surgical procedure performed in association with intraarticular ACL reconstruction. This was mainly due to the techniques that were most popular at the time, which included the use of BPTB in most cases, with reconstructions performed in acute, highly inflamed knees in an open fashion, often after diagnostic arthroscopy, followed by a very cautious rehabilitation protocol with several weeks of immobilization in a cast or brace. In these circumstances, any additional surgical procedure could have devastating effects on the joint with a high risk of arthrofibrosis and loss of range of motion (ROM), especially in extension. Basically, these techniques, even without the addition of ERs, often lead to a stiff knee rather than to a stable knee, which should be regarded as the actual goal of modern ACL surgery.

Less invasive arthroscopic-assisted techniques, the increased use of hamstring grafts and more accelerated rehabilitation have considerably reduced postoperative stiffness and arthrofibrosis, making the use of ERs less risky and more reliable.

10.2 Biomechanics

Biomechanically, ERs are justified by three main factors:

1. the longer and more efficient lever arm of structures acting on the periphery compared with the central structures in controlling rotation, such as handling a car steering wheel (Fig. 10.2). In fact, the anterolateral ligament (ALL), the most important ligament in restraining internal rotation of the knee, does not have a high ultimate failure load (175 N) and stiffness (20 N/M) because it acts from the periphery of the knee joint where less force is required [10].
2. The second factor is the protective function of ERs on the intraarticular graft, with a special emphasis on the first postoperative phase of integration and remodelling of the reconstructed ACL. This effect was first demonstrated in 1990 by Engebretsen et al. in a laboratory study where they showed a reduction in the stress applied to the ACL graft by an average of 43% [11]. The findings of Engebretsen were later confirmed by Draganich et al. [12] and more recently

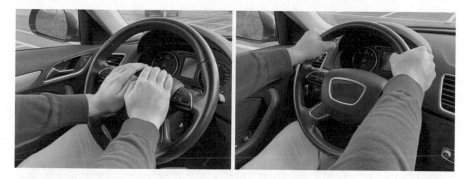

Fig. 10.2 The longer lever arm of the lateral reconstruction allows for more efficient control of tibial rotation. In this example, the steering wheel represents the tibia and the arms represent the rotational control that is exerted on it

confirmed by Marom et al. [13], who showed that LET decreased the ACL graft force up to 80% with applied pivoting loads, resulting in a better integration of the intraarticular graft as evaluated by MRI [14].

3. The third factor is that ERs aim to treat tears of secondary restraints whose injuries result in increased rotational instability and pivot shift. The biomechanical effect of an ALL tear on the rotational stability of the knee has been widely investigated in cadaveric studies [15, 16].

The biomechanical effect of ERs in controlling the pivot shift phenomenon has also been demonstrated in vivo using navigation. In a study published by our group in 2014, we evaluated the effect of the addition of an ER to intraarticular ACL reconstruction. In this study, twenty patients underwent anatomic single-bundle ACL reconstruction with doubled semitendinosus and gracilis tendons with the addition of extra-articular reconstruction. In the patients in Group A, intraarticular reconstruction was performed first, and ER was performed thereafter; in the patients in Group B, ER was performed first, and intraarticular reconstruction was performed thereafter. A navigator equipped with software designed for dynamic evaluation of the PS was used. Measurements were performed before reconstruction, after the first procedure, and after the second procedure. For the dynamic evaluation (pivot shift test), in Group A, the mean anterior tibial translation (ATT) significantly decreased from 15.0 ± 6.8 mm in the preoperative (ACL-deficient) condition to 9.4 ± 6.4 mm after ACL reconstruction and to 8.5 ± 5.4 mm after ER; the mean anterior tibial rotation (ATR) significantly decreased from 16.9° ± 4.7° to 11.6° ± 4.1° and to 6.1° ± 2.2°, respectively. In Group B, the mean ATT significantly decreased from 12.5 ± 3.3 mm in the preoperative (ACL-deficient) condition to 9.1 ± 5.9 mm after LT and to 8.1 ± 5.4 mm after ACL reconstruction; the mean ATR significantly decreased from 16.0° ± 4.5° to 9.2° ± 4.3° and to 7.5° ± 4.0°, respectively. We concluded that anatomic ACL reconstruction and EAR were synergic in controlling AP translation and the rotation of the tibia and effective in the treatment of ALRI and in reducing the pivot shift phenomenon [17] (Table 10.1.).

Table 10.1. Dynamic evaluation during the pivot shift test. In Group A, intraarticular reconstruction was performed first, followed by extra-articular reconstruction; in Group B, extra-articular reconstruction was performed first, followed by intraarticular reconstruction

Group A		Group B	
ATT, mean ± SD, mm		**ATT**, mean ± SD, mm	
ACL Deficient	14.1 ± 3.7	ACL Deficient	13.5 ± 6.5
ACL Rec	6.0 ± 1.9*	ER	10.2 ± 3.2*
ER	5.3 ± 1.6*	ACL Rec	4.0 ± 1.6*
ATR, mean ± SD, degrees		**ATR**, mean ± SD, degrees	
ACL Deficient	35.7 ± 4.8	ACL Deficient	36.7 ± 4.8
ACL Rec	28.9 ± 4.1*	ER	26.2 ± 6.2*
ER	20.9 ± 4.8*	ACL Rec	23.5 ± 4.9*

ACL anterior cruciate ligament, *ACL Rec*, anterior cruciate ligament reconstruction, *ATR* axial tibial rotation, *ATT* anterior tibial translation, *ER* extra-articular reconstruction, *SD* standard deviation. The asterisk is placed where there was a statistically significant change from the previous condition

10.3   Surgical Techniques

Surgical techniques for the treatment of anterolateral secondary restraint tears include repair techniques and reconstruction techniques.

Anterolateral complex repair is indicated only in acute cases when surgery is performed within 2 weeks of injury and the lesion is still in the inflammatory phase of healing. Furthermore, when surgery is performed acutely, the lesion of the antero-lateral aspect of the knee is easily recognized and can be better classified and repaired. In our paper published in Arthroscopy in 2017, lesions of the anterolateral complex were classified as follows: Type I: multilevel rupture with individual layers torn at different levels with macroscopic haemorrhage involving the area of the anterolateral ligament (ALL) and extended to the anterolateral capsule; Type II: multilevel rupture with individual layers torn at different levels with macroscopic haemorrhage extended from the area of the ALL and capsule to the posterolateral capsule; Type III: complete transverse tear involving the area of the ALL, usually near its insertion to the lateral tibial plateau, distal to the lateral meniscus; and Type IV: bony avulsion (Segond's fracture) [18].

As displayed in Fig. 10.3, our approach to acute lesions of anterolateral structures is to repair them, adding and retensioning the capsule to protect against the plastic elongation of the ALL and capsule occurring along with the injury. We use absorbable stitches for the repair and tensioning of the torn ligament, while we use nonabsorbable stitches and anchors only for Type 3 and 4 tears where the capsule or bony fragment need to be reapproximated and fixed to the bone.

Recently, we have also added, in some cases, a nonabsorbable suture acting as an internal brace secured to the insertion sites of the ALL on the femur and tibia to protect the repaired tissue from excessive loading during the healing phase and rehabilitation (Fig. 10.4) [19].

Using a navigation system, we evaluated the biomechanical effect of ALL repairs on patients treated acutely. Our study showed that repair of the anterolateral

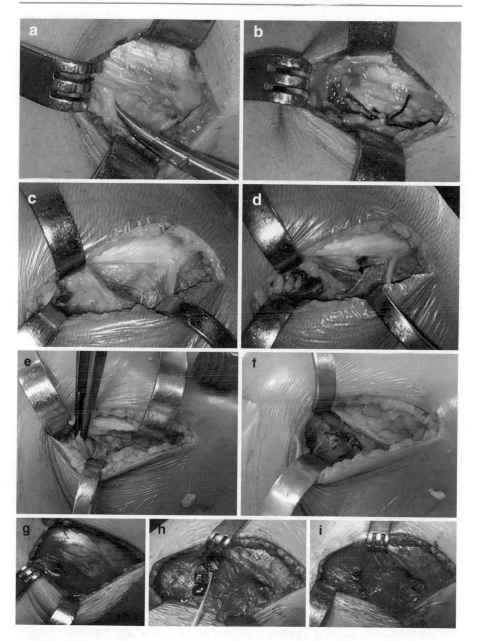

Fig. 10.3 Classification and treatment of the lesions of the anterolateral complex according to Ferretti et al. [18] (**a, b**) type I lesion; (**c, d**) type II lesion; (**e, f**) type III lesion; (**g, h, i**) type IV lesion (Segond's fracture)

Fig. 10.4 Type II lesion treated with repair/ retensioning augmented by an internal brace of the anterolateral ligament

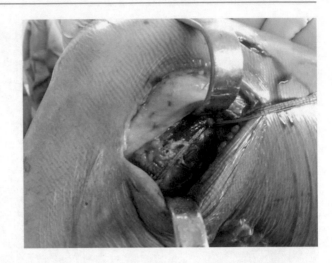

Table 10.2 Effect of ALL repair on knee stability [20]

	Before ALL and ACL surgery	After ALL surgery	After ALL and ACL surgery
Anterior tibial translation, mm	15 ± 3	11 ± 2	6 ± 3*
Axial tibial rotation, degrees	22 ± 12	16 ± 3*	10 ± 4

*$P<.05$. mm. ACL, anterior cruciate ligament; ALL, anterolateral ligament; mm, millimetres. The repair of the lateral compartment had a statistically significant effect on axial tibial rotation (ATR) ($P = .001$), with small effect on anterior tibial translation (ATT=) ($P = 0.18$). The addition of ACL reconstruction produced a significant effect on ATT ($P = .01$) with lesser, statistically nonsignificant, effect on ATR ($P = .12$)

compartment had a statistically significant effect on axial tibial rotation (Table 10.2) [20].

Reconstruction techniques can be classified into anatomical and nonanatomical techniques.

Nonanatomical techniques are basically the ERs described in the 1970s and are mostly inspired by the Lemaire technique. These techniques are all similar and based on fascia lata lateral tenodesis (LT) with or without bony fixation. The aim of these techniques is to control the internal rotation of the tibia, therefore acting on one of the two components of the PS phenomenon (rotational component). As these techniques could produce a constraint of the normal tibial internal rotation, we prefer tenodesis without bony fixation to minimize the risk of any possible overconstraint of the knee. Since the early 1980s, our preferred technique has been the modification of the Mcintosh technique proposed by Coker and Arnold [21, 22]. This is lateral tenodesis with a strip of fascia lata that is detached proximally, passed under the lateral collateral ligament, fixed to the LCL and back to Gerdy's tubercle with absorbable stitches with the knee at 90° of flexion and external rotation. This is an all-soft tissue technique with no fixation of the graft to the bone and a sort of self-adjusting mechanism throughout the ROM (Fig. 10.5).

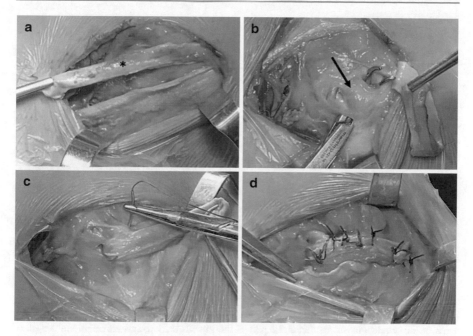

Fig. 10.5 Coker–Arnold modification of the Macintosh lateral tenodesis. The incision on the lateral side was extended to 10 to 12 cm in a hockey-stick fashion, from the Gerdy tubercle proximally to just inferior to the lateral epicondyle while the knee was flexed to 90°. (**a**) The fascia lata was exposed and incised along its fibres about 3 cm from the posterior border. With 1 cm of the iliotibial tract left intact posteriorly, a 1 cm-wide and 13-cm-long strip of the iliotibial tract was detached proximally, leaving intact its distal attachment on the Gerdy tubercle; (**b**) The lateral collateral ligament was identified, and the proximal part of the strip was passed under the ligament; (**c**) The band was then reflected on itself and sutured under tension with periosteal absorbable stitches to the Gerdy tubercle while the tibia was held in maximal external rotation; (**d**) Final appearance of the ER

Anatomical techniques are based on the description of the anatomy of the ALL as provided by Steven Claes in 2014 [23]. These techniques are based on anatomical reconstruction of the ALL by using a soft tissue graft (gracilis or strip of fascia lata) strongly fixed to the bone at the level of the anatomical insertion sites of the ALL (posterior and proximal to the lateral epicondyle on the femur and in between the fibular head and Gerdy's tubercle, 1 cm below the joint line on the tibia). One of the most popular anatomical techniques for ALL reconstruction is the one described by Sonnery-Cottet et al. in 2015 [24]. This technique consists of minimally invasive reconstruction of the ALL with a double bundle gracilis graft to reproduce the V-shaped anatomy of the ALL (Fig. 10.6).

Our preferred technique for anatomical reconstruction is the FLAT (fascia lata anterolateral tenodesis) technique described in 2016, where both layers (superficial and deep) of the anterolateral ligament, represented by the anterolateral femorotibial ligament (ALFTL) and ALL as described by Müller and Claes, respectively, are addressed (Fig. 10.7) [26].

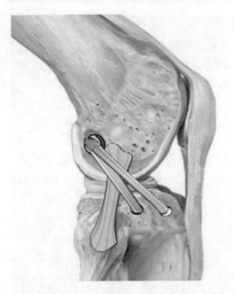
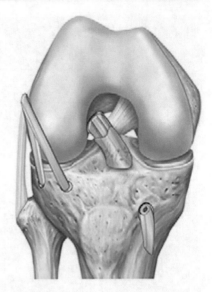

Fig. 10.6 The Sonnery-Cottet technique for ACL and ALL reconstruction. The combined graft is formed from a tripled semitendinosus tendon and gracilis tendon. The ACL graft consists of three parts of the semitendinosus tendon and 1 part of the gracilis tendon, and the additional length of the gracilis forms the ALL graft. [25]. *Courtesy of Dr. Sonnery-Cottet*

10.4   Results

As recently pointed out by Michael J. Rossi in his editorial in Arthroscopy, "Such is the case for the highly debatable anterolateral ligament (ALL) and its use as an augmentation for the anterior cruciate ligament (ACL)-deficient knee during ACL reconstruction (ACLR); the proof will be in the clinical outcome" [27]. In fact, biomechanical results are not enough to validate the efficacy of a surgical technique, as it can be demonstrated only by clinical outcomes. Therefore, only long-term follow-up clinical studies can confirm the efficacy of a surgical technique in terms of patient-reported outcomes and failure rates. In this way, it is useful to report our long experience in the field of ERs that dates back to the 1970s. These techniques were used both in isolation and in addition to an intraarticular ACL reconstruction and were based on our principles that remain unchanged today: hamstrings as graft of choice for ACL intraarticular reconstruction; out-in femoral tunnel drilling for anatomical placement of the graft; and the use of ERs when needed.

The first paper on ERs from our group was published in 1982 [28].

We treated 48 unstable knees with lateral and medial ligament plastics using the Hughston technique, which included advancement of the semimembranosus and POL on the medial side and biceps tendon on the lateral side. Thirty-six patients were athletes who had to leave their sport because of knee instability. Eight patients had a previous meniscectomy. Forty-three patients were reviewed with a follow-up of 15 to 60 months. Thirty patients were able to undertake sporting activities, but only 12 were at the top level. There were 13 surgical failures, and the results were satisfactory in approximately 50% of the cases. As a result of this quite disappointing technique, we concluded that ERs alone were not able to sufficiently stabilize the knee, especially in athletes. Therefore, since then, ERs have been used only in association with IRs. Although several ER techniques were used, such as the original Lemaire technique and the Andrews technique, we eventually selected the Coker–Arnold modification of the Macintosh technique, which is still our preferred technique due to its simplicity, reliability, and low cost. At that time, our indications for adding an ER to intraarticular ACL reconstruction were based on the grade of preoperative rotational instability as evaluated by the severity of the Jerk test and participation in high-risk sports. Over the years, we have published several papers

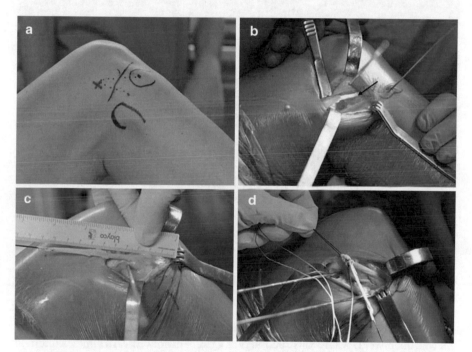

Fig. 10.7 Illustration of the FLAT technique on a left knee [26]. (**a**) Identification of the landmarks: lateral femoral epicondyle, Gerdy's tubercle, and ALL insertion at the level of the tibial plateau; measurement of the distance between them. (**b**) Identification of a central portion of the iliotibial tract (arrow); a strip is harvested in line with its fibres in a distal-to-proximal direction. (**c**) measurement of the ITB strip, left inserted at the level of the Gerdy's tubercle. (**d**) The graft is doubled and whipstitched. (**e**) The suture wire at the level of the loop is passed through the eyelet of a knotless anchor. (**f**) Measurement of the anatomic ALL bundle. (**g**) After the fixation of the first bundle on the femoral side with the knee in full extension and neutral rotation, the second bundle and tibial fixation of the graft is performed, always with the knee in full extension and neutral rotation. (**h**) Final view of the reconstruction. The first bundle (black arrow), starting from the Gerdy tubercle to the femoral insertion of the anterolateral ligament, is an anterolateral capsule reinforcement (Müller's ALFTL); the second bundle (blue arrow), fixed on the anatomic insertion points of the ALL, corresponds to the reconstructed ALL (as described by Claes et al)

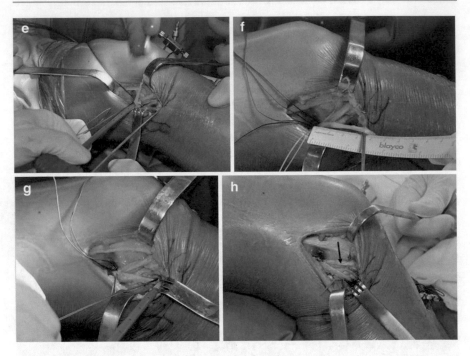

Fig. 10.7 (continued)

on this specific population composed of high-risk athletes (mainly volleyball and football athletes) with either acute or chronic ALRI [29–31].

In 1992, we published a paper on knee ligament injuries in volleyball players. This was a report of 52 professional volleyball players who underwent ACL reconstruction in our department. There were 30 acute injuries where ACL reconstruction was associated with anteromedial and/or anterolateral structure repair and 22 chronic cases where ER was added to ACL reconstruction (11 with the Andrews technique and 11 with the Coker–Arnold technique). Forty patients were available at follow-up, and 25 returned to the same level of sport [29].

In 2016, we also published a case series of 16 female professional football players who underwent ACL reconstruction plus Coker–Arnold ER. All athletes returned to the same preinjury professional level, and we had no complications or failures [32].

Another important cohort study was performed to evaluate the effectiveness of ERs, performed along with IRs, in a series of 111 cases of children and adolescents, whose results have been widely reported to be less favourable than adults and are often disappointing.

A total of 111 patients with a mean follow-up of 43.8 months were included in the study. Forty patients underwent isolated ACL reconstruction, and 71 underwent ACL reconstruction plus Coker–Arnold modification of the McIntosh technique. The addition of lateral extra-articular tenodesis to ACL reconstruction was associated with a significantly lower graft rupture rate (odds ratio 15.9, $P = .012$) than isolated ACL reconstruction and was also associated with significantly better knee stability and Tegner activity levels, with no increase in the rate of nongraft rupture-related reoperations or complications.

However, the most important paper published by our group on the long-term results of ACL reconstruction and ERs was published in Arthroscopy in 2016. We reported the results of 150 patients at a minimum of 10 years of follow-up. Seventy-five patients were treated with isolated single-bundle anatomical ACL reconstruction, and 75 were treated with ACL reconstruction plus ER. At the final follow-up, we reported similar results in the patient-reported outcome measures in the two groups, but 7 failures in the ACL reconstruction group and no failures in the ACL reconstruction plus ER group were observed. Even if at the time of surgery, ER was added for patients who showed greater rotational instability (grade 2 or 3 pivot shift), and in patients at higher risk of failure (pivot sports), the addition of ER significantly reduced the failure rate [33]. Therefore, 25 years after the Snowmass meeting, because of improvements in surgical and rehabilitation techniques, the basic biomechanical principles of AERs were successfully applied in clinical practice. In fact, in the last decade, many papers have been published that clearly demonstrate the importance of ERs, regardless of the technique used, in terms of patient satisfaction, the reduction of the failure rate, and the protection of the graft and meniscal sutures [34–36].

For this reason, it is now well recognized that the addition of ER could be indicated in cases of:

- severe rotational instability (preoperative explosive PS)
- female athletes
- high-risk athletes
- Segond's fracture
- revision surgery
- adolescents

References

1. Slocum DB, Larson RL. Rotatory instability of the knee. Its pathogenesis and a clinical test to demonstrate its presence. J Bone Joint Surg Am. 1968;50:211–25.
2. Galway HR, MacIntosh DL. The lateral pivot shift: a symptom and sign of anterior cruciate ligament insufficiency. Clin Orthop Relat Res. 1980;147:45–50.
3. Bull AMJ, Amis AA. The pivot-shift phenomenon: A clinical and biomechanical perspective. Knee; 1998.
4. Slette EL, Mikula JD, Schon JM, Marchetti DC, Kheir MM, Turnbull TL, LaPrade RF. Biomechanical results of lateral extra-articular tenodesis procedures of the knee: a systematic review. Arthroscopy. 2016;32(12):2592–611.
5. Lemaire M. Ruptures anciennes du ligament croisé antérieur. J Chir. 1967;93(3):311–20.
6. Pearl AJ, Bergfeld JA. Extra-articular reconstruction in the anterior cruciate ligament deficient knee. Snowmass: AOSSM; 1989.

7. Clancy WG, Nelson DA, Reider B, Narechania RG. Anterior cruciate ligament reconstruction using one-third of the patellar ligament, augmented by extra-articular tendon transfers. J Bone Joint Surg Am. 1982;64:352–9.
8. Getgood AMJ, Bryant DM, Litchfield R, Heard M, McCormack RG, Rezansoff A, Peterson D, Bardana D, MacDonald PB, Verdonk PCM, Spalding T, Willits K, Birmingham T, Hewison C, Wanlin S, Firth A, Pinto R, Martindale A, O'Neill L, Jennings M, Daniluk M, Boyer D, Zomar M, Moon K, Pritchett R, Payne K, Fan B, Mohan B, Buchko GM, Hiemstra LA, Kerslake S, Tynedal J, Stranges G, Mcrae S, Gullett LA, Brown H, Legary A, Longo A, Christian M, Ferguson C, Mohtadi N, Barber R, Chan D, Campbell C, Garven A, Pulsifer K, Mayer M, Simunovic N, Duong A, Robinson D, Levy D, Skelly M, Shanmugaraj A, Howells F, Tough M, Spalding T, Thompson P, Metcalfe A, Asplin L, Dube A, Clarkson L, Brown J, Bolsover A, Bradshaw C, Belgrove L, Millan F, Turner S, Verdugo S, Lowe J, Dunne D, McGowan K, Suddens CM, Declercq G, Vuylsteke K, Van Haver M. Lateral Extra-articular Tenodesis Reduces Failure of Hamstring Tendon Autograft Anterior Cruciate Ligament Reconstruction: 2-Year Outcomes From the STABILITY Study Randomized Clinical Trial. Am J Sports Med. 2020;48:285–97.
9. Amis AA. Anterolateral knee biomechanics. Knee Surg Sports Traumatol Arthrosc. 2017;25:1015–23.
10. Kennedy MI, Claes S, Fuso FAF, Williams BT, Goldsmith MT, Turnbull TL, Wijdicks CA, LaPrade RF. The Anterolateral Ligament: An Anatomic, Radiographic, and Biomechanical Analysis. Am J Sports Med. 2015;43:1606–15.
11. Engebretsen L, Lew WD, Lewis JL, Hunter RE. The effect of an iliotibial tenodesis on intraarticular graft forces and knee joint motion. Am J Sports Med. 1990;18:169–76.
12. Draganich LF, Reider B, Ling M, Samuelson M. An in vitro study of an intraarticular and extraarticular reconstruction in the anterior cruciate ligament deficient knee. Am J Sports Med. 1990;18(3):262–6.
13. Marom N, Ouanezar H, Jahandar H, Zayyad ZA, Fraychineaud T, Hurwit D, Imhauser CW, Wickiewicz TL, Pearle AD, Nawabi DH. Lateral Extra-articular Tenodesis Reduces Anterior Cruciate Ligament Graft Force and Anterior Tibial Translation in Response to Applied Pivoting and Anterior Drawer Loads. Am J Sports Med. 2020;48:3183–93.
14. Cavaignac E, Mesnier T, Marot V, Fernandez A, Faruch M, Berard E, Sonnery-Cottet B. Effect of Lateral Extra-articular Tenodesis on Anterior Cruciate Ligament Graft Incorporation. Orthop J Sport Med. 2020;8:2325967120960097.
15. Kittl C, El-Daou H, Athwal KK, Gupte CM, Weiler A, Williams A, Amis AA. The role of the anterolateral structures and the ACL in controlling laxity of the intact and ACL-deficient knee. Am J Sports Med. 2016;44:345–54.
16. Monaco E, Ferretti A, Labianca L, Maestri B, Speranza A, Kelly MJ, D'Arrigo C. Navigated knee kinematics after cutting of the ACL and its secondary restraint. Knee Surg Sport Traumatol Arthrosc. 2012;20:870–7.
17. Monaco E, Maestri B, Conteduca F, Mazza D, Iorio C, Ferretti A. Extra-articular ACL reconstruction and pivot shift: In vivo dynamic evaluation with navigation. Am J Sports Med. 2014;42:1669–74.
18. Ferretti A, Monaco E, Fabbri M, Maestri B, De Carli A. Prevalence and classification of injuries of anterolateral complex in acute anterior cruciate ligament tears. Arthroscopy. 2017;33:147–54.
19. Monaco E, Mazza D, Redler A, Drogo P, Wolf MR, Ferretti A. Anterolateral ligament repair augmented with suture tape in acute anterior cruciate ligament reconstruction. Arthrosc Tech. 2019;8:e369–73.
20. Monaco E, Ponzo A, Lupariello D, Rota P, Fabbri M, Lanzetti R, Mazza D, Ferretti A. Repair of antero lateral ligament injuries in acute anterior cruciate ligament tears: an in vivo study using navigation. Muscles Ligaments Tendons J. 2019;
21. Ireland J, Trickey EL. Macintosh tenodesis for anterolateral instability of the knee. J Bone Joint Surg Br. 1980;62:340–5.

22. Arnold JA. A lateral extra-articular tenodesis for anterior cruciate ligament deficiency of the knee. Orthop Clin North Am. 1985;16:213–22.
23. Claes S, Vereecke E, Maes M, Victor J, Verdonk P, Bellemans J. Anatomy of the anterolateral ligament of the knee. J Anat. 2013;223:321–8.
24. Sonnery-Cottet B, Thaunat M, Freychet B, Pupim BHB, Murphy CG, Claes S. Outcome of a combined anterior cruciate ligament and anterolateral ligament reconstruction technique with a minimum 2-year follow-up. Am J Sports Med. 2015;43:1598–605.
25. Saithna A, Thaunat M, Delaloye JR, Ouanezar H, Fayard JM, Sonnery-Cottet B. Combined ACL and anterolateral ligament reconstruction. JBJS Essent Surg Tech. 2018;
26. Ferretti A, Monaco E, Fabbri M, Mazza D, De Carli A. The Fascia Lata anterolateral tenodesis technique. Arthrosc Tech. 2017;6:e81–6.
27. Rossi MJ. Editorial commentary: anterolateral ligament augmentation for the anterior cruciate ligament-deficient knee debate-the proof is in the pudding. Arthroscopy. 2019;35:893–5.
28. Perugia L, Puddu G, Mariani PP, Ferretti A. Chronic anteromedial and anterolateral instability of the knee in athletes. Results of treatment with peripheral surgery. Rev Chir Orthop Reparatrice Appar Mot. 1982;68:365–8.
29. Ferretti A, Papandrea P, Conteduca F, Mariani PP. Knee ligament injuries in volleyball players. Am J Sports Med. 1992;20:203–7.
30. Ferretti A, De Carli A, Conteduca F, Mariani PP, Fontana M. The results of reconstruction of the anterior cruciate ligament with semitendinosus and gracilis tendons in chronic laxity of the knee. Ital J Orthop Traumatol. 1989;15:415–24.
31. Ferretti A, Conteduca F, De Carli A, Fontana M, Mariani PP. Results of reconstruction of the anterior cruciate ligament with the tendons of semitendinosus and gracilis in acute capsuloligamentous lesions of the knee. Ital J Orthop Traumatol. 1990;16:452–8.
32. Guzzini M, Mazza D, Fabbri M, Lanzetti R, Redler A, Iorio C, Monaco E, Ferretti A. Extraarticular tenodesis combined with an anterior cruciate ligament reconstruction in acute anterior cruciate ligament tear in elite female football players. Int Orthop. 2016;40:2091–6.
33. Ferretti A, Monaco E, Ponzo A, Basiglini L, Iorio R, Caperna L, Conteduca F. Combined intra-articular and extra-articular reconstruction in anterior cruciate ligament–deficient knee: 25 years later. Arthroscopy. 2016;32:2039–47.
34. Marcacci M, Zaffagnini S, Giordano G, Iacono F, Lo PM. Anterior cruciate ligament reconstruction associated with extra-articular tenodesis: a prospective clinical and radiographic evaluation with 10- to 13-year follow-up. Am J Sports Med. 2009;37:707–14.
35. Grassi A, Zicaro JP, Costa-Paz M, Samuelsson K, Wilson A, Zaffagnini S, Condello V. Good mid-term outcomes and low rates of residual rotatory laxity, complications and failures after revision anterior cruciate ligament reconstruction (ACL) and lateral extra-articular tenodesis (LET). Knee Surg Sports Traumatol Arthrosc. 2020;28:418–31.
36. Kandhari V, Vieira TD, Ouanezar H, Praz C, Rosenstiel N, Pioger C, Franck F, Saithna A, Sonnery-Cottet B. Clinical outcomes of arthroscopic primary anterior cruciate ligament repair: a systematic review from the scientific anterior cruciate Ligament Network International Study Group. Arthroscopy. 2020;36:594–612.

Revision ACL Reconstructions

11

Andrea Ferretti and Andrea Redler

At the beginning of modern ACL surgery dating back to the late seventies and early eighties, intraarticular ACL reconstructions were almost exclusively performed in hyperspecialized centers. Later, in the 1990s, these procedures began spreading all over the world, soon becoming one of the most frequently performed operative procedures in orthopedic surgery, as approximately 100,000 new ACL injuries occur every year in the USA alone [1].

Despite the remarkable improvements that have occurred throughout the years with regard to graft selection, tunnel placement, graft fixation, and rehabilitation and have resulted in more predictable outcomes, most studies still report a clinical failure rate between 8% and 10% for ACL reconstructions, with a peak of 25% in young and athletic populations [2]. Therefore, as the number of primary ACL reconstructions has increased, the number of revision surgeries has concurrently risen. Our experience compares well with that of more advanced sports and knee surgery clinics around the world. In our first paper on ACL revision published in the JBJS American Volume in 2006, we reported the clinical and surgical findings as well as the results of a series of 30 cases collected over seven years, from 1997 to 2003. In 2013, the number of operated cases rose to 132 [3, 4].

Failure of ACL reconstruction may be attributed to surgical technical errors, a lack of biological incorporation of the graft, a new traumatic injury, failure to address patient anatomy or the inadequate treatment of associated injuries, including tears of secondary restraints in the anterolateral compartment of the knee. While new traumatic injuries may be difficult to avoid, some modifiable, surgery-related factors, such as accuracy in reproducing native ACL anatomy and function, proper graft selection, and the appropriate treatment of all associated injuries, are key modifiable factors that may prevent ACL reconstruction failure.

A. Ferretti (✉) · A. Redler
Orthopaedic Unit, Sant'Andrea University Hospital, La Sapienza University, Rome, Italy

© The Author(s), under exclusive license to Springer Nature Switzerland AG 2022
A. Ferretti (ed.), *Anterolateral Rotatory Instability in ACL Deficient Knee*,
https://doi.org/10.1007/978-3-031-00115-4_11

Unlike primary reconstruction, revision surgery must include careful preoperative planning, which could mainly include an evaluation of possible causes of failure of the previous operation to be eventually avoided in repeated surgery. Regardless of the graft used, tunnel placement and their possible expansion as well as the presence and location of fixation devices are the most important factors to be considered. Avoiding the convergence or overlapping of the new tunnels with the previous tunnels could result in stronger fixation and faster incorporation of the graft. Fixation devices can be removed only if they actually interfere with the new tunnels, as their removal could result in significant bone loss and/or weakening of the implant site.

The use of extraarticular reconstructions in revision cases is another matter of concern. In fact, it seems likely that revisions represent the most widely accepted indication for a combined intraarticular and extraarticular procedure, as reported by most recent papers [5, 6].

Since the beginning of our practice, we carefully challenged all revision-related issues in the first rare and sporadic cases. In fact, our first well-documented ACL revision dates back to 1997.

At that time, the majority of patients who were referred to our clinic had undergone a failed nonanatomic vertically placed autograft BPTB surgery (Fig. 11.1).

Our standard, anatomic, hamstring ACL reconstruction using out-in femoral drilling was the easiest and most logical approach for all these cases, allowing us to avoid any interference with the previous femoral tunnel (Fig. 11.2).

However, the tibial tunnel and tibial fixation remained a major concern in most cases, as convergence or overlapping could never be definitely avoided. The excellent mechanical properties of the Evolgate fixation device, introduced by us in 2000 for strong tibial fixation of soft tissue grafts such as hamstrings, allowed secure

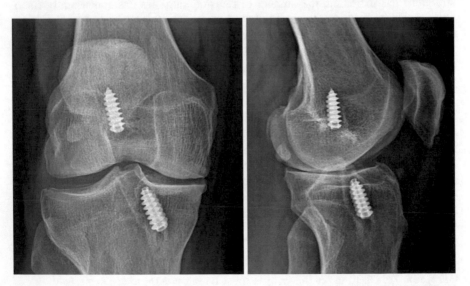

Fig. 11.1 Failure of a single incision nonanatomical vertically placed BPTB graft (Rosenberg's technique)

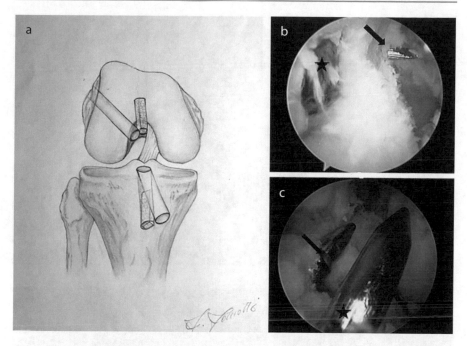

Fig. 11.2 (a) Independent drilling of the tunnels; the out-in technique often avoids any interference with a previous femoral tunnel (courtesy of Ferdinando Iannotti). Fig **b** shows the previous femoral tunnel incorrectly placed anterior to the resident ridge (black star); the tip of the K guide wire is placed in the anatomical femoral footprint of the ACL, just in front of the over-the-top position (black arrow). Fig. **c** shows an incorrect anterior tibial tunnel (black star), while the black arrow indicates the new tibial tunnel

fixation even in cases of significant bone loss or exit tunnel convergence [7]. The Evolgate is a fixation device that comprises three components, all made of titanium alloy: a coil (a spiral that is 21 mm long and 10 mm in diameter) with a spike positioned at one extremity, a 9 X 20 mm screw, and a washer (Figs. 11.3 and 11.4).

Before the tendons are pulled through the tibial tunnel, the spiral is inserted into the tibial tunnel with a dedicated impactor, which also provides penetration of the spike in the predrilled tibial cortex. After the tendons are pulled through the bone tunnels and secured to the femoral side, the ends of the four tendons coming out of the tibial tunnel are properly tensioned. The screw and the washer are then inserted, interfering with the tendons and the spiral until the washer is pressed against the tibial cortex. The spike prevents the rotation of the spiral as the screw tightens. The reinforcement of the tunnel walls and the use of a large, threatened interference screw provide very strong and stiff fixation, as documented by several biomechanical studies [7, 8].

Regarding femoral fixation, our preference is to use a suspension device (Swing Bridge), which offers strong and stiff fixation by means of its cortical grip (Fig. 11.5). Moreover, after the final fixation of both sides (tibial and femoral), the Swing Bridge

Fig. 11.3 The Evolgate is formed by three components: a coil with a spike on the top (A) and a screw with a washer on the extremity

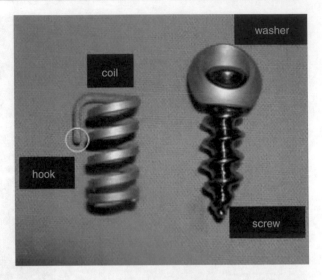

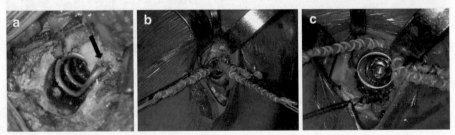

Fig. 11.4 Tibial fixation of the free ends of the hamstrings by the Evolgate. (**a**) A coil fixed into the tibial tunnel (black arrow indicates the hook); (**b**) tendons coming out from the tunnel; (**c**) definitive fixation by a screw and washer

allows a final adjustment of the tension of the reconstructed ACL by a simple rotation of the device (Fig. 11.5a).

As stated before, previous fixation devices should be removed to avoid any interference with the new drilled tunnel. The removal of fixation devices could result in bone loss, possibly weakening the site of fixation.

Accurately checking the actual position of the fixation devices preoperatively and properly planning the site and direction of the new tunnels could allow most of the previous fixation devices to be kept in place during the revision surgery (Fig. 11.6).

Nonaggressive postoperative rehabilitation was used in all cases. The knee was placed in a full extension brace for 2–3 weeks with weight-bearing as tolerated with crutches. Progressive range of motion exercises were then encouraged. At 5–6 weeks, the use of the brace was discontinued, and weight-bearing without crutches was permitted. A muscle strengthening program was prescribed for two to

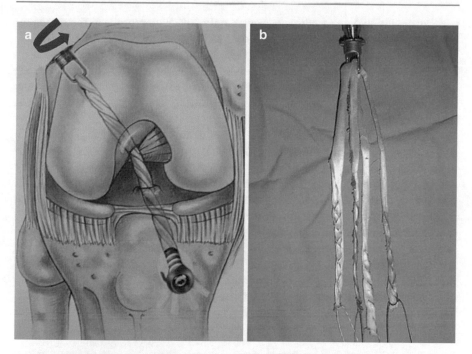

Fig. 11.5 (a) Femoral cortical fixation: In addition to providing excellent strength, the use of the swing bridge allows the new ligament to be retensioned, even after tibial fixation, by further screwing it (**a**. Red arrow) Reprinted with permission from Citieffe catalog, Bologna, Italy). Figure **b** shows the gracilis and semitendinosus tendons doubled on the swing bridge

four months after surgery, and a gradual return to athletic training was allowed between 4 and 6 months postoperatively.

In our 2006 paper, we presented the surgical technique and the results of a series of twenty-eight out of thirty consecutive patients who underwent a revision ACL with double semitendinosus and gracilis tendon grafts combined with an extraarticular stabilizing procedure [9]. Primary ACL reconstruction was performed elsewhere with the use of BPTB grafts in 26 patients and with a prosthetic ligament in four patients. The average time from the primary reconstruction to the revision was five years (range one to eleven years). The same surgical technique was used in all cases (arthroscopic-assisted two incision anatomic hamstrings reconstruction along with an extraarticular reconstruction with the fascia lata according to the McIntosh technique as modified by Coker and Arnold). In four patients, a two-stage procedure was performed because of difficulties encountered in the removal of pre-existing fixation devices, which resulted in excessive bone tunnel enlargement. Two-stage procedures date back to before Evolgate fixation was introduced. In addition to the reconstructive procedure, six lateral and three medial partial meniscectomies were performed.

At follow-up, the mean subjective and objective ISAKOS score was 84 +- 12, with 15 patients categorized as A, 11 as B, 2 as C, and none as D. All but one patient was satisfied with the procedure. However, only 20% had returned to the same pre-injury sport and level and 30% had returned to the same sport but at a lesser level.

The overall rate of failure was 10% (three out of the twenty-eight revisions).

Encouraged by the early results of our surgical approach to ACL revisions, we continued using this technique, extending the use of hamstrings (harvested from the contralateral side) to cases of failure of previous ipsilateral hamstring ACL reconstruction.

Our preliminary experience with the use of contralateral hamstrings in revision ACL surgery was published in 2011 [10]. The paper reported the results, at a minimum follow-up of two years, of twelve consecutive cases of revision ACL surgery collected between 2005 and 2008, where contralateral hamstrings were used as ACL grafts along with extraarticular (Coker–Arnold) reconstruction. The most important finding of this study was that at follow-up, the ability to return to work and resume sport activities as well as subjective knee function and knee stability were significantly improved. The results were in line with the most satisfactory outcomes reported in the literature. Using a grade 2 or 3 pivot shift and/or a KT1000 side-to-side difference >5 mm as the definition of failure, only one failure was recorded (8.4%). As donor site morbidity could be a major concern in cases of tendon harvesting from the contralateral healthy knee, it was carefully assessed at follow-up. In our

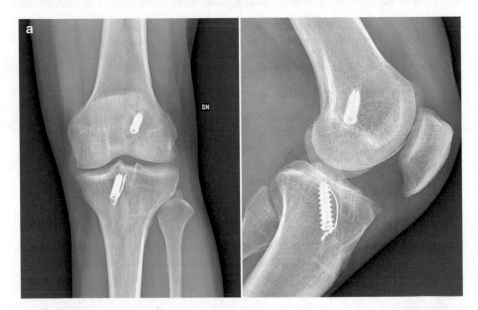

Fig. 11.6 (a) Preoperative X-ray of a failed BPTB ACL reconstruction. The tibial fixation device could interfere with the new tunnel. (b) To avoid screw removal, a new tibial tunnel was drilled just tangential to the previous tunnel (tunnel scope showing the threads of the previously implanted interference screw). (c) Emergence of the tibial tunnel in the anatomic ACL footprint. (d) The Evolgate spiral is positioned, occupying the distal half of the tibial tunnel. (e) Proper positioning of an adequately tensioned DGST graft. (f) Postoperative X-ray showing the old and new fixation devices

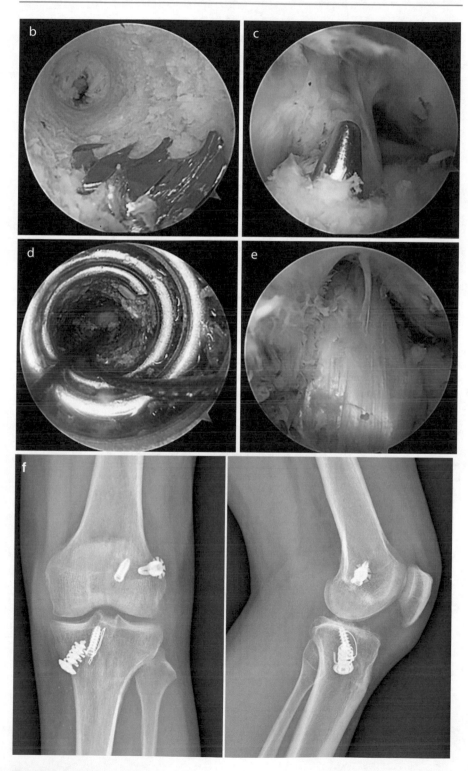

Fig. 11.6 (continued)

series, tendon harvesting was performed using the standard technique with a commercially available tendon stripper without a tourniquet. There was no need for a brace or specific rehabilitation, while weight-bearing was allowed postoperatively as tolerated. No complications were observed, and at the subjective evaluation, no patient complained of problems at the harvested site, with the Lysholm score and IKDC subjective score at the time of follow-up being 100 for all patients.

Our overall experience with the use of hamstrings combined with a lateral extraarticular procedure in revision ACL reconstructions was comprehensively presented in the 2018 paper published in Arthroscopy, where we reviewed 118 out of the 132 patients operated on at our institution with a mean follow-up of more than ten years (3–19 years) from 1997 to 2013. At follow-up, the patients demonstrated a significant improvement in patient-reported outcomes and clinical and arthrometric results compared with the preoperative evaluation (Table 11.1.).

At the objective evaluation, the patients had significantly improved in stability testing with no cases of reduced range of motion. Nine patients had >5 mm side-to-side differences on the KT-1000 or 2+ pivot shift tests and were considered failures (<8%). All patients in this series returned to their daily life activities. Of these patients, 49 (41.5%) returned to their desired type and level of sport; however, 31 (26.3%) preferred less stressful activity for reasons other than the operated knee. Thirty-eight (32.2%) returned to the same sport but at a lower level.

We speculate that the low rate of failure observed in this series was due to the addition of lateral extraarticular reconstruction to intraarticular reconstruction. In fact, revision surgery is currently considered the most recognized indication for adding lateral tenodesis to the intraarticular graft [11].

Table 11.1. Clinical and arthrometric results

	Preoperative evaluation	Follow-up evaluation	T test
Tegner score (SD)	3.6 ± 1.8	5.7 ± 1.9	$P < 0.0001$
Lysholm score (SD)	66.98 ± 19.8	90.0 ± 7.2	$P < 0.0001$
IKDC subjective score (SD)	70.3 ± 8.4	85.7 ± 12.3	$P < 0.0001$
IKDC objective score			
A	0	53 (45.0)	$P < 0.0001$
B	0	56 (47.5)	
C	36 (30.5)	9 (7.5)	
D	82 (69.5)	0 (0)	
Pivot Shift grade, n (%)			
Negative/0	0 (0)	82 (69.5)	$P < 0.0001$
1+ (glide)	26 (22)	32 (27.1)	
2+ (clunk)	51 (43.2)	4 (3.4)	
3+ (sublux)	41 (34.7)	0 (0)	
KT-1000, mm	7.2 ± 2.6	2.2 ± 1.6	$P < 0.0001$
KT-1000, n (%)			
<3 mm	0	61 (51.7)	$P < 0.0001$
3–5 mm	19	48 (40.6)	
>3 mm	99	9 (7.7)	

The rate of osteoarthrosis after an ACL injury and reconstruction is another area of intense research, with a high number of young patients developing degenerative joint diseases after ACL reconstruction, regardless of the type of reconstruction performed [9, 12]. Furthermore, the rate of osteoarthrosis after revision ACL reconstruction appears to be higher than the rate reported after primary ACL reconstruction, even when similar techniques of combined intraarticular and extraarticular reconstructions are used. In our study, the radiological evaluation at follow-up demonstrated signs of severe degenerative joint diseases in 25% of cases. This high prevalence of radiological signs of osteoarthrosis may be explained by the sheer number of instability episodes leading to ACL failures and the higher rate of chondral and meniscal tears encountered in revision cases, which was reported to be as high as 70% in our series. In fact, meniscectomy is considered the most important factor affecting radiological worsening and clinical outcomes in ACL-deficient and reconstructed knees.

In recent years, the use of accelerated rehabilitation has become the standard after ACL reconstruction. However, it is well known that biological secure fixation and tendon-to-bone healing require at least twelve weeks [13]. Therefore, accelerated rehabilitation and the related micromotion of the graft inside the tunnels could compromise the bone tendon interface, resulting in poor biological fixation [14]. When hamstring grafts are used, especially in revision cases, and even when strong and stiff fixation devices are used, we believe that a slower rehabilitation program, such as the one employed in our studies, is beneficial [3].

In conclusion, revision ACL reconstruction with doubled semitendinosus and gracilis combined with extraarticular reconstruction provides continued improvement in clinical outcomes at mid- to long-term follow-up. Meniscectomy, which is often required, is the main factor related to worsened radiological signs of degenerative osteoarthritis.

References

1. Gianotti SM, Marshall SW, Hume PA, Bunt L. Incidence of anterior cruciate ligament injury and other knee ligament injuries: a national population-based study. J Sci Med Sport. 2009;12:622–7.
2. Wright RW, Gill CS, Chen L, et al. Outcome of revision anterior cruciate ligament reconstruction: a systematic review. J Bone Joint Surg Am. 2012;94:531–6.
3. Ferretti A, Conteduca F, Monaco E, De Carli A, D'Arrigo C. Revision anterior cruciate ligament reconstruction with doubled semitendinosus and gracilis tendons and lateral extraarticular reconstruction. J Bone Joint Surg Am. 2006;88(11):2373–9. https://doi.org/10.2106/JBJS.F.00064. PMID: 17079393.
4. Redler A, Iorio R, Monaco E, Puglia F, Wolf MR, Mazza D, Ferretti A. Revision anterior cruciate ligament reconstruction with hamstrings and extra-articular tenodesis: a mid- to long-term clinical and radiological study. Arthroscopy. 2018;34(12):3204–13. https://doi.org/10.1016/j.arthro.2018.05.045. Epub 2018 Oct 3. PMID: 30292594.
5. Trojani C, Beaufils P, Burdin G, et al. Revision ACL reconstruction: influence of a lateral tenodesis. Knee Surg Sports Traumatol Arthrosc. 2012;20:1565–70.
6. Ventura A, Legnani C, Boisio F, Borgo E, Peretti GM. The association of extra-articular tenodesis restores rotational stability more effectively compared to contralateral hamstring tendon

   autografts ACL reconstruction alone in patients undergoing ACL revision surgery. Orthop
   Traumatol Surg Res. 2021;107(2):102739.
 7. Ferretti A, Conteduca F, Morelli F, Ticca L, Monaco E. The Evolgate: a method to improve
    the pullout strength of interference screws in tibial fixation of anterior cruciate ligament recon-
    struction with doubled gracilis and semitendinosus tendons. Arthroscopy. 2003;19:936–40.
 8. Ferretti A, Conteduca F, Labianca L, Monaco E, De Carli A. Evolgate fixation of doubled
    flexor graft in anterior cruciate ligament reconstruction: biomechanical evaluation with cyclic
    loading. Am J Sports Med. 2005;33(4):574–82.
 9. Rothrauff BB, Jorge A, de Sa D, Kay J, Fu FH, Musahl V. Anatomic ACL reconstruction
    reduces risk of post-traumatic osteoarthritis: a systematic review with minimum 10-year fol-
    low-up. Knee Surg Sports Traumatol Arthrosc. 2020;28(4):1072–84.
10. Ferretti A, Monaco E, Caperna L, Palma T, Conteduca F. Revision ACL reconstruction using
    contralateral hamstrings. Knee Surg Sports Traumatol Arthrosc. 2013;21:690–5.
11. Shybut TB. Editorial commentary: this is the way: extra-articular augmentation is an
    essential consideration in contemporary anterior cruciate ligament surgery. Arthroscopy.
    2021;37(5):1667–9. https://doi.org/10.1016/j.arthro.2021.01.014. PMID: 33896515.
12. Ferretti A, Monaco E, Ponzo A, Basiglini L, Iorio R, Caperna L, Conteduca F. Combined
    intra-articular and extra-articular reconstruction in anterior cruciate ligament-deficient knee:
    25 years later. Arthroscopy. 2016;32(10):2039–47.
13. Gulotta LV, Rodeo SA. Biology of autograft and allograft healing in anterior cruciate ligament
    reconstruction. Clin Sports Med. 2007;26(4):509–24.
14. Vadalà A, Iorio R, De Carli A, Argento G, Di Sanzo V, Conteduca F, Ferretti A. The effect
    of accelerated, brace free, rehabilitation on bone tunnel enlargement after ACL recon-
    struction using hamstring tendons: a CT study. Knee Surg Sports Traumatol Arthrosc.
    2007;15(4):365–71.

Anterolateral Instability and Osteoarthrosis

Andrea Ferretti, Fabio Conteduca, Raffaele Iorio, and Edoardo Viglietta

Since Allmann, as reported by De Haven, defined anterior cruciate ligament (ACL) tears as "the beginning of the end of the knee" in the sixties [1], the close interaction between ACL tears and degenerative osteoarthritis (DOA) has been a matter of intensive study and great debate. In fact, Allmann referred to the cascade of events related to ACL insufficiency, such as meniscal and cartilage tears leading to DOA, as occurring almost inevitably as a result of instability (Figs. 12.1 and 12.2).

As a consequence of Allmann's statement, in addition to recovering knee stability and function, most surgeons recommended ACL surgery with the aim of preventing DOA.

Our interest in DOA in ACL-deficient and reconstructed knees dates back to the late eighties, when the first operated patients became available for a medium-term follow-up, which was adequate enough for a reliable evaluation of the eventual progression of DOA. Some of these very early studies, mainly based on our pioneering experience in ACL reconstruction, are worthy of reporting, as their conclusions, somehow original and futuristic, were later fully confirmed by almost all following studies on this matter and are still relevant today.

The first study [2], published in 1991 in AJSM after the usually long pathway of submission, revisions, and resubmission, investigated the effect of long-lasting ACL insufficiency and related instability on the knee, with a special focus on cartilage tears. By retrospectively evaluating a series of 500 medical records of patients undergoing an open procedure for ACL insufficiency, 162 (32%) showed chondromalacia to some extent. Factors that significantly increased the rate of chondral damage were previous surgeries failing to stabilize the joint (meniscectomies), the time from the first injury to surgery with a peak when this time exceeded 24 months,

A. Ferretti (✉) · F. Conteduca · R. Iorio · E. Viglietta
Orthopaedic Unit, Sant'Andrea University Hospital, La Sapienza University, Rome, Italy

© The Author(s), under exclusive license to Springer Nature Switzerland AG 2022
A. Ferretti (ed.), *Anterolateral Rotatory Instability in ACL Deficient Knee*, https://doi.org/10.1007/978-3-031-00115-4_12

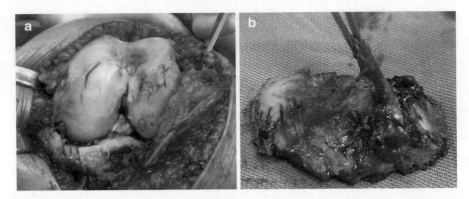

Fig. 12.1 Surgical finding of knee osteoarthritis in a 57-year-old male 26 years after undergoing ACL reconstruction with a hamstring autograft (**a**). The tibia was cut with a semitendinosus graft still successfully integrated (**b**)

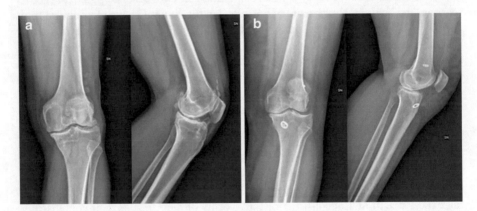

Fig. 12.2 Radiological evidence of severe degenerative osteoarthritis (DOA) of the knee. (**a**) Anteroposterior and lateral X-ray views of the knee of a 62-year-old male 26 years after undergoing ACL reconstruction. (**b**) Anteroposterior and lateral X-ray views of the knee of a 60-year-old female 23 years after undergoing ACL reconstruction

the level of sports participation, and the degree of rotatory instability (Pivot Shift ++ or +++) (Figs. 12.3, 12.4 and 12.5).

In a subsequent paper [3], published only a few months later but reporting more extensive and reliable experience, the progression of DOA was evaluated five years after ACL reconstruction with hamstrings in a series of 114 patients. The prevalence of radiological signs of DOA, as described by Fairbank [4], was statistically correlated with meniscectomies performed at the time of reconstruction. As the number of meniscectomies performed in acute cases was significantly lower than that performed in chronic cases, the timing of reconstruction was also correlated with the severity of DOA. A definite, but not statistically significant, correlation was also found between residual rotational instability as revealed by a clinically detectable jerk test at follow-up and radiological signs of DOA (Tables 12.1 and 12.2).

Fig. 12.3 Rate of
chondromalacia and the
time from the initial injury
to surgery for each level of
sport participation

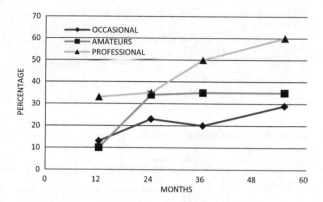

Fig. 12.4 Rate of
chondromalacia and the
time from the initial injury
to surgery

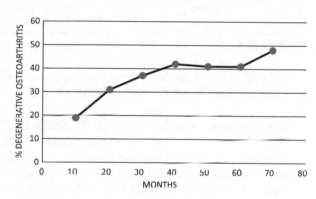

Fig. 12.5 Chondromalacia
and the severity of the
pivot shift test

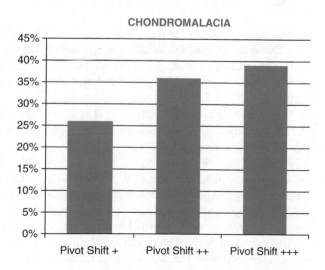

As a result, the protective effect of the operative stabilizing procedure could be effective only if reconstruction was performed before an irreparable meniscal tear eventually occurred as a result of ACL deficiency.

Table 12.1 Meniscectomies performed in acute and chronic ACL-deficient knees

	Acute ACL tear (55 knees)	Chronic ACL tear (59 knees)	p value
Medial	11 (20%)	35 (59%)	p < 0.05
Lateral	7 (13%)	6 (10%)	p < 0.05
Both menisci	2 (3%)	4 (7%)	p < 0.05
Total	20 (36%)	45 (76%)	p < 0.05

Table 12.2 Radiological changes following ACL reconstruction with and without meniscectomy

Fairbank gradings	Meniscectomies 65 knees (100%)	No meniscectomies 49 knees (100%)	p value
0	17 (26%)	29 (59%)	p < 0.05
1	24 (37%)	15 (31%)	Ns
2-4	24 (37%)	5 (10%)	p < 0.05

Ns not significant

Therefore, the conclusions of our older papers on the interactions between ACL tears and DOA can be summarized as follows:

- Knee instability, resulting from ACL deficiency, almost inevitably causes cartilage and meniscal tears, leading to degenerative changes up to osteoarthrosis.
- Meniscal tears and eventual meniscectomy represent the real point of no return since degenerative changes rapidly progress towards osteoarthrosis.
- ACL reconstructions are unable to fully preserve the joint from degenerative changes, which inevitably occur to some extent.

ACL reconstruction can be somewhat effective in preventing DOA whether surgery is able to stabilize the joint before irreparable meniscal tears eventually occur.

In the following years, many papers have been published on this issue, with results almost perfectly matched the conclusions we presented several decades earlier.

In a systematic review, in 2019, Mehel et al. [5] concluded that chronic instability in ACL-deficient knees is associated with a significant increase in medial meniscus injuries after six months, followed by a significant increase in cartilage lesions after 12 months, therefore recommending early surgery within 12 months after the initial ACL injury. In 2015, Brambilla et al. [6], on the basis of a retrospective review of 988 patients whose medical records were retrospectively investigated, concluded that the risk of developing at least one associated meniscal or cartilage lesion increases by an average of 0.6% for each month of delay of surgical reconstruction.

The same conclusions were reported in a study by Anderson and Anderson [7], where they correlated the prevalence of meniscal and cartilage injuries in children and adolescents with the timing of ACL reconstruction. Both studies recommended early surgical intervention to prevent meniscal and cartilage injuries. The role of meniscectomy in the development of DOA after ACL reconstruction was also emphasized in a meta-analysis by Ruano et al. [8], which extensively confirmed the previous findings of Claes et al. [9], who had already stated that some degree of DOA is inevitable as a consequence of ACL reconstruction and that an associated meniscal resection dramatically increases the risk of developing DOA.

Kessler et al. [10], based on a long-term follow-up of 136 ACL reconstruction, stated that *"the risk of secondary meniscal tears is reduced after ACL reconstruction, which reduces the negative effects of DOA after surgery."*

The findings of these recent studies reveal how brilliant and forward-thinking the conclusions of our 30-year-old studies were.

All these studies, as well as many others, mainly dealt with the interaction between ACL-deficient knees, ACL reconstructions, and degenerative changes without specifically focusing on the role of extra-articular reconstructions (EARs) in the development of DOA.

However, this is a crucial point because degenerative changes, early radiological signs of DOA, and a reduced postoperative range of motion (ROM) could be a result of EAR-related overconstraint of the knee. The risk of overconstraint is the main concern for most surgeons who are still hesitant to regularly adopt EARs.

As an attempt to remove some of the perplexity and bewilderment related to possible overconstraint resulting from EARs, only the analysis of long-term studies of patients who underwent ACL reconstructions with or without EARs as an adjunct could be conclusive.

In the study published in Arthroscopy [11] in 2017, we reported the clinical and radiological findings of two groups of patients who underwent anatomic ACL reconstruction with hamstrings alone or with a modified extra-articular McIntosh procedure as described by Arnold–Cocker, which were reviewed after a minimum follow-up of eleven years. Comparing the two groups in terms of radiological signs of DOA, as evaluated using the Fairbank, Kellegren and IKDC scales, no increased sign of DOA was observed in the group of patients who underwent the combined procedure in either the tibiofemoral or patellofemoral joints. In contrast, in two out of the three scales, a statistically significant lower degree of DOA was detected in the group where EAR was added (Fig. 12.6).

In the further revision of many of the same patients, the results reviewed at a longer follow-up of 15 years were quite similar, with an obvious symmetric light progression of radiological signs in both groups. In this investigation, the effect of EARs on the lateral compartment of the knee, likely more involved by overconstraint, was assessed. Neither the overall tibiofemoral joint nor the lateral compartment of the knee showed higher DOA development. Rather, in the case of partial lateral meniscectomy, combined ACL reconstruction may have a protective effect against the premature development of DOA (Figs. 12.7 and 12.8) (Tables 12.3 and 12.4).

This issue had already been investigated by Pierpaolo Mariani, another fellow of Professor Perugia, who suggested performing open capsular retensioning in cases of partial lateral meniscectomy for professional soccer players. This simple procedure avoids subtle rotatory instability, and the related high risk of cartilage damage and chondrolysis eventually occurs in the lateral compartment of the knee [12].

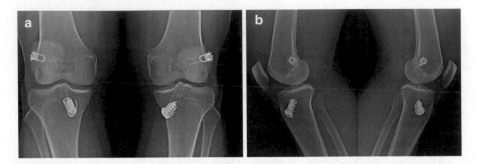

Fig. 12.6 Anteroposterior (**a**) and lateral (**b**) weight bearing X-rays of knees after combined bilateral ACL reconstruction plus EAR performed 18 years and 14 years earlier for the right and left knee, respectively. No meniscectomy was performed at any time. Radiological signs of DOA were absent

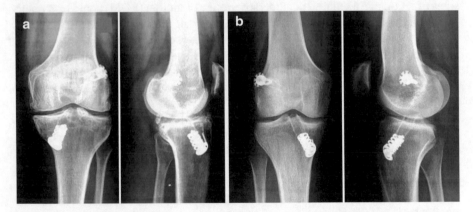

Fig. 12.7 Radiological evidence of DOA after ACL reconstruction. (**a**) A 46-year-old male 17 years after undergoing isolated ACL reconstruction without meniscectomy; (**b**) A 43-year-old male 16 years after undergoing combined ACL reconstruction plus EAR without meniscectomy

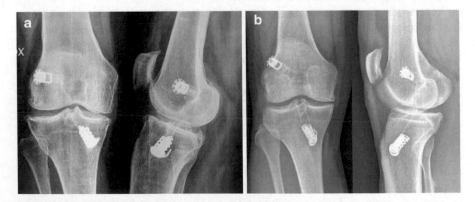

Fig. 12.8 Radiological evidence of DOA of the lateral compartment of the knee after ACL reconstruction and partial lateral meniscectomy. (**a**) A 49-year-old male 18 years after undergoing partial lateral meniscectomy and isolated ACL reconstruction; (**b**) A 45-year-old male 18 years after undergoing partial lateral meniscectomy and combined ACL reconstruction plus EAR

Table 12.3 Overall tibiofemoral compartment radiological results: Comparison between isolated ACLR and combined ACLR and EAR with a minimum follow-up of 15 years

Overall tibiofemoral joint	Lateral tibiofemoral joint				Medial tibiofemoral joint	
15 years follow-up	Isolated ACLR (79 pts)	ACLR+ EAR (76 pts)	Isolated ACLR (79 pts)	ACLR+ EAR (76 pts)	Isolated ACLR (79 pts)	ACLR+ EAR (76 pts)
IKDC score	*p* = 0.01		*p* = 0.03		*p* = 0.98	
Group A	40 (50.63%)	41 (53.95%)	40 (50.63%)	51 (67.11%)	29 (36.71%)	17 (22.37%)
Group B	25 (31.65%)	31 (40.79%)	28 (35.44%)	22 (28.94%)	27 (34.18%)	37 (48.68%)
Group C	13 (16.45%)	2 (2.63%)	10 (12.66%)	3 (3.95%)	19 (24.05%)	19 (25%)
Group D	1 (1.27%)	2 (2.63%)	1 (1.27%)	–	4 (5.06%)	3 (3.95%)
FAIRBANK classification	*p* = 0.94		*p* = 0.22		*p* = 0.78	
Grade I	36 (45.57%)	38 (50%)	30 (37.97%)	38 (50%)	12 (15.19%)	10 (13.16%)
Grade II	27 (34.17%)	23 (30.26%)	34 (43.04%)	29 (38.16%)	33 (41.77%)	35 (46.05%)
Grade III	13 (16.46%)	13 (17.11%)	12 (15.19%)	9 (11.84%)	25 (31.65%)	22 (28.95%)
Grade IV	3 (3.80%)	2 (2.63%)	3 (3.80%)	–	9 (11.39%)	9 (11 84%)
KELLGREN classification	*p* = 0.04		*p* = 0.04		*p* = 0.61	
Grade 0	9 (11.39%)	8 (10.53%)	15 (18.99%)	37 (48.68%)	7 (8.86%)	5 (6.58%)
Grade I	38 (48.10%)	49 (64.47%)	31 (39.24%)	19 (25%)	19 (24.05%)	23 (30.26%)
Grade II	19 (24.05%)	13 (17.10%)	20 (25.31%)	15 (19.74%)	35 (44.30%)	31 (40.79%)
Grade III	11 (13.92%)	5 (6.58%)	13 (16.46%)	5 (6.58%)	13 (16.46%)	12 (15.79%)
Grade IV	2 (2.54%)	1 (1.32%)	–	–	5 (6.33%)	5 (6.58%)

To date, by carefully reviewing the small number of studies investigating the development of DOA in ACL reconstructed knees, there is no evidence that adding EAR to intra-articular reconstruction would result in an increased rate of DOA over time. Moreover, as any reduction in ROM has never been reported as a result of EAR, we can reasonably conclude that lateral tenodesis does not result in any clinically relevant risk of overconstraint.

Based on our experience and the review of the current literature, our conclusions can be more extensively summarized as follows:

- ACL tears result in knee instability, which generates cartilage and meniscal tears over time.
- These injuries progressively worsen and lead to osteoarthrosis.

Table 12.4 Lateral tibiofemoral compartment radiological results: Comparison between lateral meniscectomy and no meniscectomy performed with isolated ACLR and combined ACLR and EAR with a minimum follow-up of 15 years

15 years follow-up	Isolated ACLR		ACLR + EAR	
	Lateral meniscectomy *(16 pts)*	No meniscectomy *(63 pts)*	Lateral meniscectomy *(12 pts)*	No meniscectomy *(64 pts)*
IKDC score	**p = 0.60**		**p = 0.40**	
Group A	8 (50%)	32 (50.79%)	6 (50%)	45 (70.31%)
Group B	4 (25%)	24 (38.10%)	5 (41.67%)	17 (26.56%)
Group C	4 (25%)	6 (9.52%)	1 (8.33%)	2 (3.13%)
Group D	–	1 (1.59%)	–	–
FAIRBANK classification	**p = 0.03**		**p = 0.69**	
Grade I	5 (31.25%)	25 (39.68%)	6 (50.00%)	32 (50%)
Grade II	5 (31.25%)	29 (46.03%)	5 (41.67%)	24 (37.50%)
Grade III	5 (31.25%)	7 (11.11%)	1 (8.33%)	8 (12.50%)
Grade IV	1 (6.25%)	2 (3.18%)	–	–
KELLGREN classification	**p = 0.70**		**p = 0.19**	
Grade 0	2 (12.50%)	13 (20.63%)	6 (50.00%)	31 (48.44%)
Grade I	8 (50%)	23 (36.51%)	1 (8.33%)	18 (28.13%)
Grade II	1 (6.25%)	19 (30.16%)	4 (33.34%)	11 (17.18%)
Grade III	5 (31.25%)	8 (12.70%)	1 (8.33%)	4 (6.25%)
Grade IV	–	–	–	–

- Sports-related overuse increases the prevalence and severity of degenerative changes.
- Although the worsening of degenerative changes usually develops very slowly, it can suddenly accelerate as a result of meniscectomy whenever performed as a result of irreparable meniscal tears.
- The prevalence of meniscal tears, although quite rare in acute cases, becomes common in chronic cases.
- ACL reconstruction, either associated with stable meniscal repair or performed before an irreparable meniscal tear has occurred, is often able to preserve menisci, therefore slowing joint degeneration.
- ACL reconstruction should be performed as early as possible, especially for athletes, whose activity plays an important role in the development of DOA.
- EARs performed along with intra-articular reconstructions do not result in any increased risk of osteoarthrosis; in contrast, by contributing to rotational stability, they can protect menisci, either healthy or repaired, as well as cartilage, especially in cases of lateral meniscectomies [13].
- To date, there is no proof of any clinically relevant overconstraint of the knee resulting from the extensive use of EAR.

References

1. De Haven KE. Arthroscopy in the diagnosis and management of Anterior Cruciate Ligament deficient knee. Clin Orhtop Rel Res. 1983;172:52–6.
2. Conteduca F, Ferretti A, Mariani PP, Puddu G, Perugia L. Chondromalacia and chronic anterior instabilities of the knee. Am J Sports Med. 1991;19(2):119–23.
3. Ferretti A, Conteduca F, De Carli A, Fontana M, Mariani PP. Osteoarthritis of the knee after ACL reconstruction. Int Orthop. 1991;15(4):367–71.
4. Fairbank TJ. Knee joint changes after meniscectomy. J Bone Joint Surg. 1984;30B:664–70.
5. Mehl J, Otto A, Baldino JB, Achtnich A, Akoto R, Imhoff AB, Scheffler S, Petersen W. The ACL-deficient knee and the prevalence of meniscus and cartilage lesions: a systematic review and meta-analysis (CRD42017076897). Arch Orthop Trauma Surg. 2019;139(6):819–41.
6. Brambilla L, Pulici L, Carimati G, Quaglia A, Prospero E, Bait C, Morenghi E, Portinaro N, Denti M, Volpi P. Prevalence of associated lesions in anterior cruciate ligament reconstruction: Correlation with surgical timing and with patient age, sex, and body mass index. Am J Sports Med. 2015;43(12):2966–73.
7. Anderson AF, Anderson CN. Correlation of meniscal and articular cartilage injuries in children and adolescents with timing of anterior cruciate ligament reconstruction. Am J Sports Med. 2015;43(2):275–81.
8. Ruano JS, Sitler MR, Driban JB. Prevalence of radiographic knee osteoarthritis after anterior cruciate ligament reconstruction, with or without meniscectomy: an evidence-based practice article. J Athl Train. 2017;52(6):606–9.
9. Claes S, Hermie L, Verdonk R, Bellemans J, Verdonk P. Is osteoarthritis an inevitable consequence of anterior cruciate ligament reconstruction? A meta-analysis. Knee Surg Sports Traumatol Arthrosc. 2013;21(9):1967–76.
10. Kessler MA, Behrend H, Henz S, Stutz G, Rukavina A, Kuster MS. Function, osteoarthritis and activity after ACL-rupture: 11 years follow-up results of conservative versus reconstructive treatment. Knee Surg Sports Traumatol Arthrosc. 2008;16(5):442–8.
11. Ferretti A, Monaco E, Ponzo A, et al. Combined intra-articular and extra-articular reconstruction in anterior cruciate ligament–deficient knee: 25 years later. Arthrosc J Arthrosc Relat Surg. 2016;32(10):2039–47.
12. Mariani PP, Garofalo R, Margheritini F. Chondrolysis after partial lateral meniscectomy in athletes. Knee Surg Sports Traumatol Arthrosc. 2008;16(6):574–80.
13. Sonnery-Cottet B, Saithna A, Blakeney WG, Ouanezar H, Borade A, Daggett M, Thaunat M, Fayard JM, Delaloye JR. Anterolateral ligament reconstruction protects the repaired medial meniscus: a comparative study of 383 anterior cruciate ligament reconstructions from the SANTI Study Group with a minimum follow-up of 2 years. Am J Sports Med. 2018;46(8):1819–26.

Clinical Results in ACL Surgery

13

Andrea Ferretti, Federico Morelli, and Matteo Guzzini

The first intraarticular ACL reconstruction with the semitendinosus was performed in our Hospital by Giancarlo Puddu in November 1979, using an original technique of distal detachment with a bone plug [1] (Fig. 13.1a, b). Soon thereafter the technique was definitively set up by adding the gracilis tendon harvested from the pes anserinus, along with the semitendinosus in the same bone plug.

As a result of very encouraging results, all the charts of the operated patients, including all the sequential follow-up, were collected to more comprehensively evaluate the clinical outcomes, possible complications, and return to sports activities.

In 1986, when no well-recognized rating system specifically addressed the evaluation of knee function and clinical outcomes after ACL reconstruction had been published, Puddu et al. [2], proposed a method to evaluate results of ACL reconstruction.

In this preliminary study, the evaluation of patients included both subjective and objective criteria.

Subjectively the patients were asked about pain, hydrarthrosis, and giving way (absent, rare and only sports related, frequently sports related and frequent). Patient's satisfaction at follow-up was graded as very satisfied, satisfied, somehow disappointed, and disappointed.

Objectively the knee was assessed by evaluating the range of motion and stability (Lachman test and Jerk test graded as −,+,++,+++).

A rating system was eventually set up on a scale up to 100 points, where for all subjective and objective criteria were graded as positive or even negative scores (Table 13.1).

The return to sports was evaluated separately by assigning a "sports value" to each knee according to the type and level (Table 13.2) where a maximum value of

A. Ferretti (✉) · F. Morelli · M. Guzzini
Orthopaedic Unit, Sant'Andrea University Hospital, La Sapienza University, Rome, Italy

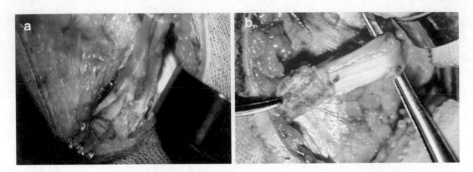

Fig. 13.1 (**a, b**) Identification of the bone insertion of semitendinosus and gracilis tendon (**a**). Harvesting of the bone plug including both semitendinosus and gracilis insertion (**b**)

Table 13.1 Results evaluation sheet. Patients scoring 90–100 points are evaluated as very good results, 75–89 point as good results, 74–50 as fair results, and <50 points as poor results

Subjective results					
Satisfaction		Pain		Giving way	
	Points		Points		Points
Very satisfied	15	Never	10	Never	20
Satisfied	10	Occasional after effort	5	Occasional during sport	5
Disappointed	5	Occasional	0	Occasional in daily activity	0
Very disappointed	0	Frequent after effort	−5	Frequent during sport	−10
				Frequent in daily activity	−20
Objective results					
Jerk		Lachman		Hydrarthrosis	
	Points		Points		Points
−	20	−	10	Never	10
+	10	+	0	Occasional after effort	5
++	−10			Occasional	0
+++	−20			Frequent after effort	−5
				Frequent	−10
		Range of motion			
		Full ROM points 15			
Loss of flexion				**Loss of extension**	
	Points				Points
<130°	5			<9°	0
<120°	−10			10°–19°	−20
<110°	−30			>20°	−30

50 points was given to a professional high-risk sport player and a minimum of 5 points was given to a patient who was not involved in any sports activity.

As soon as clinical results become reliable and adequate follow-up was obtained in an acceptable series of patients, a series of studies on clinical results of the Puddu's technique were eventually published.

Table 13.2 Sports value of the knee

Sport level	Points
Professional	
High risk	50
Middle risk	35
Low risk	20
Amateur	
High risk	45
Middle risk	30
Low risk	15
Week-end	
High risk	30
Middle risk	15
Low risk	10
Sedentary	
	5

In the first paper [3] published in 1988, among the 127 patients with anterolateral and/or anteromedial knee instabilities who were surgically treated between 1979 and 1983, 108 were reviewed and/or interviewed at a mean follow-up of 5 years (range 4–7). In all patients, ACL reconstruction was performed using the distally detached semitendinosus tendon and advancement of the biceps tendon (see Fig. 1.4) was always added laterally; when medial meniscectomy was performed, advancement of the posterior oblique ligament and semimembranosus tendon was also added (see Fig. 1.2).

According to the previously published rating system, among the 88 athletes reviewed, there were 37 very good, 39 good, and 12 fair or poor results (13.6%). The Lachman test was fully negative in 67% of the patients and frankly positive in 22%; the jerk test was negative in 64%, + in 28% and ++ in 8% of the patients. Full range of motion was recovered by 95% of the patients. The return to sport at the preinjury level was referred by only 60% of the patients, but only 20% of the patients ascribed failure to return to sport to the operated knee (instability or apprehension).

The authors concluded that the results of ACL reconstruction with the semitendinosus associated with biceps tendon advancement and semimembranosus and POL advancement in cases of medial meniscectomy were considered to be satisfactory overall but amendable.

In a subsequent paper [4], the same group evaluated the clinical results of a series of 88 patients with chronic anterolateral instability out of a group of more than 300 patients who underwent ACL reconstruction with the semitendinosus and gracilis tendon between 1982 and 1986; in all cases, lateral tenodesis was added (29 cases of the Andrews technique and 59 of McIntosh technique as modified by Coker and Arnold).

At a mean follow-up of 41 months (range 24–73), the patients were reevaluated according to the same previously published rating system. There were 43 (49%) very good results, 29 (33%) good results, 15 (17%) fair results, and 1 (1%) poor

Table 13.3 Clinical results in patients with and without meniscectomy

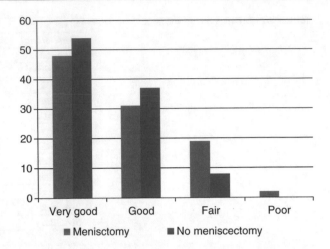

■ Menisctomy   ■ No meniscectomy

result. Seventy-one percent of the patients presented a negative Jerk test, 27% presented positive +, and 2% presented positive ++. Full range of motion was achieved in 91% of the patients and 96% were very satisfied or satisfied.

Meniscectomy associated with ACL reconstruction resulted in a lower rate of satisfactory (very good and good) results (Table 13.3).

In conclusion, the proposed technique was considered safe and effective but prolonged postoperative immobilization and its related long rehabilitation were evaluated as problematic issue.

One year later, in 1990 [5], 55 cases of acute ACL tears that were surgically treated within ten days of the initial injury were reviewed with a mean follow-up of 50 months (range 28 to 81) and clinically evaluated as previously reported. The ACL was reconstructed with only the semitendinosus in 20 cases and with the semitendinosus and gracilis in 35 cases according to Puddu's technique. In 32 cases, the remnant of the ACL, when possible, was used for augmentation. Fourteen cases of severe injuries of the medial compartment and 17 of the lateral compartment were found and surgically treated by repair. In 10 cases, lateral tenodesis (Andrews or Coker–Arnold technique) was added. Postoperative treatment included cast immobilization in flexion for 6 weeks followed by cautious rehabilitation.

At follow-up, 96% of the overall results were satisfactory (41 very good and 10 good). In 43 patients, the Jerk test was negative, and in 10, it was positive +. Full range of motion was recovered in all but one patient. However, due to a delay in recovering range of motion in 10 cases a manipulation under general anesthesia was performed at three months postoperatively.

Due to the lower number of irreparable meniscal tears and meniscectomies performed compared with a group of patients with chronic anterolateral instability operated in the same period, the authors concluded that early surgery in cases of acute ACL tears be recommended whenever possible. However, the risk of postoperative knee stiffness and arthrofibrosis should be considered and possibly adequately assessed.

As a former volleyball player and team doctor of the Italian National Volleyball team for several years, I have always been (the main author) interested in volleyball injuries. In the AJSM in 1992, we published a report on 52 volleyball players, selected among the 1041 patients operated who underwent ACL reconstruction from 1979 to 1989 [6]. The sample consisted of 10 men and 42 women. Being that the number of registered men and female volleyball players is almost the same in Italy, this statistically significant difference led to the conclusion that, given the same risk exposure, women are more subjected to ACL injuries than men. At that time, this was quite a new statement. Among the 40 players with an adequate follow-up of two years, 26 returned to preinjury sports, one of them at a lesser level, after 11 months on average. For the first time a new device, specifically designed to measure jumping ability (Bosco Ergo Jump) was used as a means to quantitatively assess the essential physical performance for the investigated sport. In either the squat jump or counter movement jump tests, the difference between operated and unaffected legs was minimal and statistically nonsignificant.

In all these papers, the results of the original Puddu's technique were presented. In summary, 85% to 90% of the results obtained overall were satisfactory. However, the price of the postoperative pain and immobilization and the prolonged and often painful rehabilitation was eventually considered unacceptable. Since the early 1990s, several changes in the surgical technique were introduced, but basic principles such as the use of hamstrings and anatomic placement of the graft by out-in femoral drilling and the use of extra-articular reconstruction remained unchanged.

In 2001, after a successful clinical trial, new very reliable fixation devices for femoral and tibial fixation of a double hamstrings free graft (Swing Bridge and Evolgate) become commercially available and become our preferred fixation devices for either primary or revision ACL reconstruction.

In 2010 [7] the first extensive report on the results of this ACL reconstruction technique was published based on the results of a series of one hundred patients who underwent a minimum follow-up of five years. In all patients, arthroscopically assisted two incision ACL reconstruction with hamstrings was performed along with extra-articular reconstruction according to Coker and Arnold in case of severe rotatory instability and high-risk athletes (23/100). Cortical fixation to the bone was achieved on the femur using the Swing Bridge and, the tibia using the Evolgate. Postoperative rehabilitation was standardized for all patients: the operated knee was placed in a full extension brace for two weeks with weight bearing on crutches as tolerated. Progressive range of motion exercises were then encouraged. At six weeks postoperatively, full weight bearing without brace was permitted. From two to four months postoperatively, a muscle strengthening program was prescribed, and between four to six months a gradual return to specific sports training was encouraged.

At the final follow-up, eight patients were lost and eighty returned for comprehensive clinical and radiological valuation. Eleven patients were evaluated only by telephone interview.

No statistically significant difference was found in the clinical results when comparing acute and chronic cases, patients with or without meniscectomy, and patients with or without extra-articular reconstruction. However, considering as biomechanical failure a pivot shift test graded as ++ or +++ and/or a KT 1000 maximum manual side-to-side difference > 5mm, six patients were found (3 men and 3 women) all of them operated on without extra-articular tenodesis.

Tunnel enlargement was radiologically measured with the method described by L'Insalata et al. [8]; in the present series, a 4.3% widening of the tunnel was found on the femoral side and a 16.9% widening was found on the tibial side; however, the widening exceeded 25% of the original side in only one patient. The limited tunnel enlargement observed in the present series could be attributed to either the stiffness of fixation devices (preventing slippage and micromovements) or initially cautious rehabilitation [9] which, however, did not prevent patients from returning to their pre-operative level of activity within six months postoperatively.

The highly satisfactory results obtained in this series show that anatomic single bundle ACL reconstruction with double semitendinosus and gracilis tendons by out-in femoral drilling is a safe and effective procedure in stabilizing ACL-deficient knee. Moreover, the combination of intraarticular and extra-articular procedures is a valid option to restore rotatory instability in medium-term follow-up, especially in severe rotatory instabilities and high-risk athletes.

Thanks to the collaboration of the team doctor of the Women Italian National Football team, a special focus was given to athletes at particular risk [10]. Sixteen elite (professional or semiprofessional) female football players were operated on between January 2007 and December 2010 for an acute (within 14 days) ACL-deficient knee. All patients underwent the same surgical procedure: anatomical ACL reconstruction with an autologous semitendinosus tendon along with extra-articular reconstruction (Coker–Arnold modified McIntosh procedure, Fig. 13.2) [4].

At follow-up, the results were excellent (87.1 IKDC subjective score; 10 patients with class A and 6 with class B IKDC objective scores) and regarding knee stability, only 1 patient showed a side-to-side maximum manual difference between 3 and 5 and no patient exceeded 5mm; only 2 patients reported a positive + – – pivot shift test with no patients with + + – or + + +. All players were able to resume football at the preinjury level and were still active at the time of the latest follow-up (72.6 ± 8.1 months). In addiction to the reliability of the surgical technique performed early, a few days after injury, this surprisingly high rate of success obtained in this series of athletes at high risk could be explained by the strong motivation of elite athletes who have easy access to any rehabilitation facilities (see Fig. 9.13).

The treatment of acute ACL tears is still controversial as many authors recommend delayed operation due to the increased risk of postoperative complications such as knee stiffness and arthrofibrosis, therefore only recommending early surgery in selected cases of professional athletes.

In our practice, we divide ACL tears into three phases: acute (within 2 weeks since initial trauma), subacute (from two weeks to complete recovery of full range of motion, usually gained within 6 weeks after proper rehabilitation), and chronic (full range of motion, painless knee).

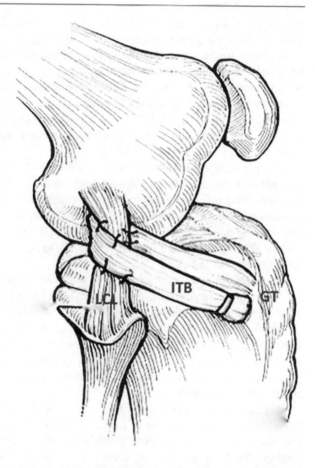

Fig. 13.2 Extra-articular reconstruction according to McIntosh as modified by Cocker Arnold. *LCL* Lateral collateral ligament, *GT* Gerdy's tubercle, *ITB* ileo-tibial band (reprinted with permission from reference # 10)

On the basis of our experience, surgery should be safely performed in acute (as soon as possible and in any case no later two weeks) or chronic cases, with the sub-acute phase being the riskiest for postoperative complications and problematic rehabilitation.

One of our students, Alessandro Giuliani, has recently presented a graduation thesis focused on the results of early ACL reconstruction performed within two weeks since initial trauma [11].

Taking advantage of the pathway designed by the chief of our Emergency Department to provide early hospitalization, MRI and eventual surgery to all young and active patients clinically diagnosed with a recent ACL tear, the author collected a series of one hundred patients who underwent operations between November 2013 and February 2019. All patients received anatomic (out-in) ACL reconstruction with double semitendinosus and gracilis tendons along with the repair and/or reconstruction of the antero-lateral ligament (ALL). Preoperatively there were 74 men and 26 women, with a mean age of 25.6 ± 10.4 years, who were all involved in various sports activities. At surgery, in addiction to ACL intraarticular reconstruction, repair/retensioning of the ALL was performed in 53 patients, reconstruction was performed in 47 patients according to Coker and Arnold. Postoperatively the knee was placed in a full extension brace with weight bearing allowed with crutches as tolerated. Beginning in the first week, the patient were instructed to remove the brace several times a day and encouraged to progressively bend the knee to reach 90° of flexion within two weeks. Rehabilitation then progressed as usual.

All patients were retrospectively evaluated at a minimum follow-up of one year (mean 39 months, range 12–78) and a complete physical examination was performed using the IKDC scale, Tegner and Lysholm score, and Knee Injury and Osteoarthritis Outcome Score (KOOS).

Comprehensively the results showed excellent results (Table 13.4). Only two patients showed unsatisfactory results being in class C in the IKDC Objective scale and presenting a side-to-side maximum manual difference > 5mm. No major complications occurred and manipulation under anesthesia was not required to recover full range of motion in any case. A non-statistically significant trend towards better results in the group where reconstruction of the ALL was added to simple repair/retensioning was found.

Based on this study, our approach to acute ACL tears, addressing early surgery for all young and active patients whose activities likely require good knee stability, is strongly supported and encouraged.

Another population at higher risk of ACLR failure, regardless of the technique used, are children, adolescents, and teenagers as a higher rate of graft rupture and recurrent instability has been documented by many authors [12, 13].

The use of combined IR and ER has been suggested to reduce the rate of failure in this specific population.

Recently we conducted a study aimed to compare the clinical outcomes of isolated ACLR versus combined ACLR+Extra-articular tenodesis young patients hypothesizing that the combined procedure would result in a lower rate of failure. A retrospective analysis of a consecutive series of pediatric and adolescent patients (aged under 18) who underwent ACLR with or without the Coker–Arnold modification of the McIntosh procedure was conducted [14]. Clinical outcomes including the graft ruptures rate, patient reported outcomes measures (KOOS and subjective IKDC) knee stability, the return to sports rate, re operations, and complications

Table 13.4 Clinical results in acute ACL reconstruction

Subjective evaluation		Clinical evaluation	
	Average		Patients (%)
KOOS	92.6 ± 6.4	*Lachman test*	
Symptoms	89.1 ± 9.6	−	82
Pain	93.2 ± 8.8	+	16
ADL	98.2 ± 3.8	++	2
Sport/Rec	85.6 ± 14.1	*Pivot shift test*	
QoL	82.7 ± 16.2	−	74
TLKSS	93.3 ± 7.0	+	24
IKDC	90.4 ±8.2	++	2
		+++	0

were assessed. One hundred and eleven patients of a mean age of 16.2 ± 1.5 years (range 13–17.6) were reviewed at a mean follow-up of 43.8 months (range 24–89). Forty patients underwent isolated ACLR and 71 underwent ACLR +LET. The addition of LET to ACLR was associated with a significant lower graft rupture rate, with significant better stability and Tegner activity level scores. There were no significant difference exceeding known minimal clinically important difference (MCID) thresholds with respect to any other outcomes measures evaluated, and no differences in the rate of non-graft rupture related reoperations or complications between the groups. We therefore concluded that combined ACLR and LET has significant advantages over isolated ACLR in pediatric and adolescent patients. These advantages include a significant reduction in graft ruptures and better knee stability with no increase in the rate of non-graft rupture related reoperations or complications.

However, the most important and comprehensive study where the role of extra-articular reconstruction, used along with IR, in the treatment of ACL-deficient knee and ALRI was carefully investigated was published in Arthroscopy in 2016 [15]. The study was conducted 25 years after the Snowmass AOSSM consensus conference, which result in ERs being almost completely given up as risky and unuseful procedures.

In this study, two groups of 75 ACL-deficient patients underwent ACLR with hamstrings with or without extra-articular reconstruction between 2002 and 2003 were reviewed and carefully clinically and radiographically evaluated at a long-term follow-up of a minimum of 10 years. The group of patients where LET was added included patients with a higher risk of graft failure (severe pivot shift, high risk sports).

At follow-up subjective scores improved significantly in both groups with no significant difference. Objectively, the number of patients receiving C and D IKDC objective activity scores in the IR alone group was significantly higher than that in the IR+ER group. Considering a side-to-side arthrometric difference more than 5 mm, a pivot shift test graded as ++ or +++, or any giving way episode occurring postoperatively as a failure, we found 8 cases in the IR group and no case in the IR+ER group ($p = .01$), despite the IR group not including high-risk patients. Radiologic evaluation showed fewer degenerative arthritic changes in the IR+ER group in both the tibiofemoral and patellofemoral joints.

Based on the results of this study, adding ER to an arthroscopically assisted anatomically placed IR, followed by modern rehabilitation protocol, does not increase the risk of postoperative degenerative osteoarthritis and may be able to improve postoperative knee stability and reduce rate of failure.

The results of this study were consistently confirmed by another, more recent, paper published in the AJSM where the role of ER was also deeply investigated, with a special focus on radiographic evidence of signs of degenerative osteoarthritis [16]. In this paper 165 cases of ACLR with or without ER were reviewed at an even longer follow-up of 15 years.

In this study, patients undergoing isolated ACLR experienced a higher risk of developing DOA than those who also underwent LET. Concurrent and subsequent partial meniscectomy were the main risk factors that were negatively associated with radiological changes in DOA. Additionally, patients undergoing the combined procedure continued to present better knee stability and a lower graft ruptures rate at a very-long-term follow-up.

References

1. Puddu G. Method for reconstruction of the anterior cruciate ligament using the semitendinosus tendon. Am J Sports Med. 1980;8(6):402–4.
2. Puddu G, Mariani P, Ferretti A, Conteduca F. Chronic anterior laxity of the knee: classification and coding of the results of surgical treatment. Ital J Orthop Traumatol. 1986;12(2):167–78.
3. Puddu G, Ferretti A, Conteduca F, Mariani P. Reconstruction of the anterior cruciate ligament by semitendinosus transfer in chronic anterior instability of the knee. Ital J Orthop Traumatol. 1988;14(2):187–93.
4. Ferretti A, De Carli A, Conteduca F, Mariani PP, Fontana M. The results of reconstruction of the anterior cruciate ligament with semitendinosus and gracilis tendons in chronic laxity of the knee. Ital J Orthop Traumatol. 1989;15(4):415–24.
5. Ferretti A, Conteduca F, De Carli A, Fontana M, Mariani PP. Results of reconstruction of the anterior cruciate ligament with the tendons of semitendinosus and gracilis in acute capsulo-ligamentous lesions of the knee. Ital J Orthop Traumatol. 1990;16(4):452–8.
6. Ferretti A, Papandrea P, Conteduca F, Mariani PP. Knee ligament injuries in volleyball players. Am J Sports Med. 1992;20:2.
7. Ferretti A, Monaco E, Giannetti S, Caperna L, Luzon D, Conteduca F. A medium to long-term follow-up of ACL reconstruction using double gracilis and semitendinosus grafts. Knee Surg Sports Arthrosc. 2011;19:473–8.
8. L'Insalata JC, Klatt B, Fu FH, et al. Tunnel expansion following anterior cruciate ligament reconstruction: a comparison of hamstring and patellar tendon autografts. Knee Surg Sports Traumatol Arthrosc. 5:234–8.
9. Vadalà A, Iorio R, De Carli A, Argento G, Di Sanzo V, Conteduca F, Ferretti A. The effect of accelerated brace free, rehabilitation on bone tunnel enlargement after ACL reconstruction using hamstring tendon: a CT study. Knee Surg Sports Arthrosc. 2007;15:365–71.
10. Guzzini M, Mazza D, Fabbri M, Lanzetti R, Redler A, Iorio C, Monaco E, Ferretti A. Extra-articular tenodesis combined with an anterior cruciate ligament reconstruction in acute anterior cruciate ligament tear in elite female football players. Int Orthop. 2016; ISSN 0341-2695
11. Giuliani A, Monaco E, Ferretti A. Acute treatment of ACL ruptures: a mid-term follow up study. Graduation thesis Sapienza University; 2020.
12. Webster KE, Feller JA. Exploring the high reinjury rate in younger patients undergoing anterior cruciate ligament reconstruction. Am J Sports Med. 2016;44(11):2827–32.
13. Wiggings AJ, Grandhi RK, Schneider DK, Stanfield D, Webster KE, Myer GD. Risk of secondary injury in younger athletes after anterior cruciate ligament reconstruction. Am J Sports Med. 2016;44(7):1861–76.
14. Monaco E, Carrozzo A, Saithna A, Conteduca F, Annibaldi A, Marzilli F, Minucci M, Sonnery-Cottet B, Ferretti A. Adolescent patient experience significantly lower ACL graft rupture rates when ACL reconstruction is combined with the Arnold-Coker modification of the MacIntosh lateral extra-articular tenodesis. Am J Sports Med. In press
15. Ferretti A, Monaco E, Ponzo A, Basiglini L, Iorio R, Caperna L, Contedca F. Combined intra-articular and extra-articular reconstruction in anterior cruciate ligament- deficient knee: 25 years later. Arthroscopy. 2016;32(10):2039–47.
16. Viglietta E, Ponzo A, Monaco E, Iorio R, Drogo P, Andreozzi V, Conteduca F, Ferretti A. ACL reconstruction combined with the Arnold-Coker modification of the MacIntosh lateral extra-articular tenodesis: long-term clinical and radiological outcomes. Am J Sports Med. 2021; in press. 2022;50(2):404–14.

Future Directions: ACL Repair vs Reconstruction

14

Andrea Ferretti, Edoardo Monaco,
and Alessandro Annibaldi

Anterior cruciate ligament reconstruction represents one of the most performed surgical procedures worldwide, with very good results in terms of restoring knee stability, recovering function, and returning to sports at the preinjury level.

Although substantial differences still exist among surgeons regarding the type of reconstruction (autologous, homologous or allografts) and graft choice in the case of autologous grafting, there is consensus that when surgery is needed, ACL reconstruction is the gold standard, as ACL repair is considered unreliable.

However, in the last few years, the number of papers on direct repair of ACL published in the international literature has increased, showing a growing interest in this topic. It appears that ACL repair should be reconsidered as an alternative to reconstruction, taking advantage of new surgical materials, devices and techniques.

Even in this case, repair is not a new concept since, as Latins used to say, "nihil sub sole novi" (nothing new under the sun).

In fact, ACL repair was the first procedure ever reported in the history of ACL surgery, although the reported results of this pioneering surgery were never trustworthy. Since the beginning of modern ACL surgery, dating back to the 1960s, the results of ACL repair, as reported by many authors over the years, were unsatisfactory overall, with few exceptions [1–4], leading knee surgeons to conclude that a torn ACL was irreparable.

Nevertheless, a deep study of the biological basis regulating the different healing phases of human ligaments reveals that even the ACL seems to have the potential to heal through different phases (Figs. 14.1, 14.2, 14.3 and 14.4) [5–7].

The blood supply, whose anatomy was also investigated by an Italian researcher [8], is rich in vessels and anastomoses providing supply to all kinds and sites of tears (proximal, distal, midsubstance). The early platelet clot seems to be able to deliver

A. Ferretti (✉) · E. Monaco · A. Annibaldi
Orthopaedic Unit, Sant'Andrea University Hospital, La Sapienza University, Rome, Italy

A. Ferretti (ed.), *Anterolateral Rotatory Instability in ACL Deficient Knee*,
https://doi.org/10.1007/978-3-031-00115-4_14

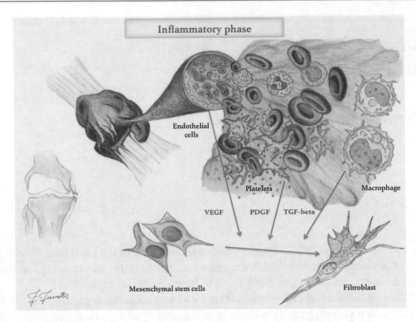

Fig. 14.1 Ligament healing. Phase I Inflammation. After injury, platelets provide a provisional clot and deliver growth factors that attract circulating and endothelial mesenchymal cells, also governing their differentiation towards fibroblasts. (Courtesy of Ferdinando Iannotti)

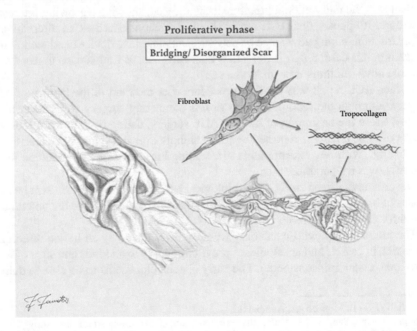

Fig. 14.2 Ligament healing: Phase II Proliferation. (Courtesy of Ferdinando Iannotti). Fibroblasts produce tropocollagen filaments and collagen fibres. A disorganized fibrous bridge replaces the provisional clot, resulting in a more substantial but still mechanically unreliable bridge (scar tissue)

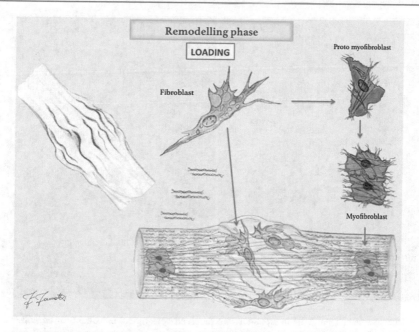

Fig. 14.3 Ligament healing. Phase III. Remodelling (Courtesy of Ferdinando Iannotti). Loading governs the progressive orientation of fibres along the axis of the ligament, and myofibroblasts could help the ligament to gain its original length and tension

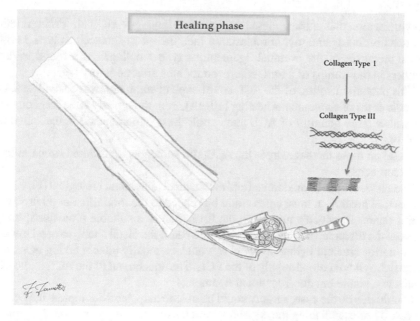

Fig. 14.4 Ligament healing. Phase IV. Definitive healing. Provisional collagen 3 is replaced by definitive collagen 1, resulting in a fully repaired and mechanically stable ligament. (Courtesy of Ferdinando Iannotti)

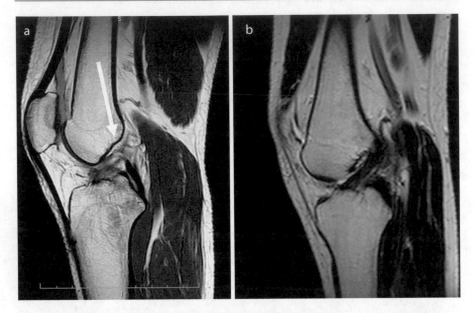

Fig. 14.5 Sagittal T2W MRI in a patient who received nonsurgical treatment for an ACL injury. (**a**) MRI conducted at the time of the ACL rupture (arrow); (**b**) MRI conducted 7 months after the injury showing an isointense signal of the ACL compared to the PCL, showing possible healing of the torn ACL

growth factors that attract mesenchymal cells and govern their differentiation towards fibroblasts and myofibroblasts. In fact, these cells, as well as type 3 collagen, a precursor of the eventual ligamentous type 1 collagen, are found in large numbers in the stumps of a torn ACL, even months after an injury [9].

This potential healing of the ACL could explain some reports of small series or sporadic cases of spontaneous healing [10–12], even though any knee surgeon dealing with a large quantity of ACL tears could have experienced similar outcomes (Fig. 14.5).

Based on these factors, why is the ACL still somehow considered irreparable by many surgeons?

The answer could be anatomical and mechanical rather than biological (Fig. 14.6). The lack of healing in most cases could be related to the intraarticular environment of this ligament, which could avoid the formation of a suitable provisional bridge between the disrupted stumps. Gravity would cause the distal stump to bend towards the posterior cruciate ligament where it would eventually attach, taking advantage of the rich synovial blood supply of the PCL. The attachment of the ACL to the PCL results in a viable but non-functional ligament.

Should this be the case, surgery could be able to help nature complete the healing process by re-establishing the continuity and tension of the ligament early, promoting scar tissue formation and differentiation.

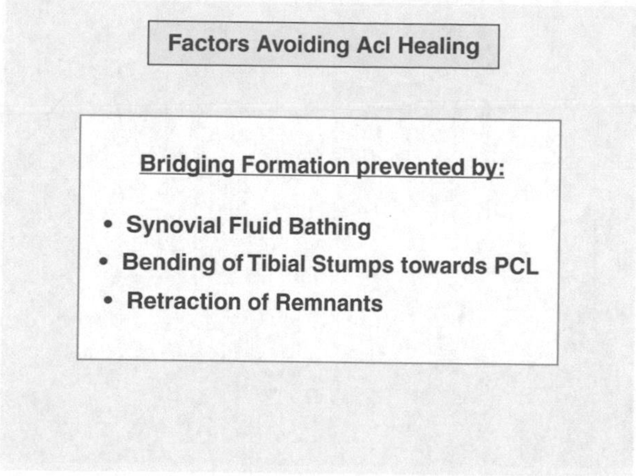

Fig. 14.6 Factors
preventing ACL healing

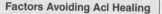

> **Factors Avoiding Acl Healing**
>
> **Bridging Formation prevented by:**
>
> - **Synovial Fluid Bathing**
> - **Bending of Tibial Stumps towards PCL**
> - **Retraction of Remnants**

It is likely that unsuccessful ACL repair attempts, as reported in the past, could be related to inaccurate patient selection, rougher and more invasive surgical techniques performed through open arthrotomies, inappropriate material, prolonged postoperative immobilization and old-fashioned rehabilitation protocols.

Encouraged by some reliable and trustworthy papers [13–15] and based on solid biological concepts, we reconsidered ACL repair as a possible alternative to reconstruction in selected cases a few years ago.

After some successful attempts, in our hospital, a new project was started in January 2018 that aimed to perform surgical repairs of acute ACL tears in adults whenever technically possible. All patients referred to our emergency department with a clinically proven acute, complete, ACL tears and who were to undergo operations within two weeks of their injury were provisionally selected for a prospective study.

At surgery, based on their arthroscopic appearance, the tears were classified according to the site and type of injuries as suggested by Sherman et al. [16].

Site of injury: I: proximal, close to the roof; II: midsubstance, with a tibial stump longer than 50%; III: midsubstance, with a tibial stump shorter than 50%; and IV: distal, close to tibial insertion.

Tissue quality: A: compact stump, very firm; B: moderately fringed stump, holding sutures; and C: severely fringed stump, not holding sutures (Fig. 14.7).

Type IA, IB, IIA and IIB injuries were considered repairable and were repaired. Patients with other types of injuries underwent standard ACL reconstruction with hamstrings (Fig. 14.8).

Surgical technique of ACL repair by a transosseous pull-out suture of the tibial stump over the lateral femoral condyle.

The patient was set to undergo a standard knee procedure. A transtendinous portal was used for diagnostic arthroscopy, and the anteromedial portal was used as a working portal. The torn ACL was carefully evaluated and probed to identify the

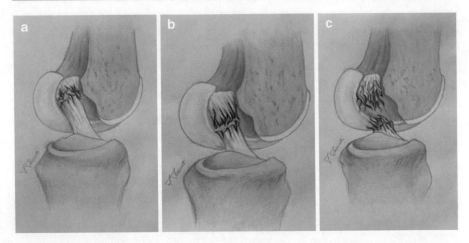

Fig. 14.7 Examples of tears of the anterior cruciate ligament: (**a**) grade I-A, proximal tear with a very firm stump and/or only a mildly frayed end; (**b**) grade II-B, midsubstance proximal (<50%) tear with a moderately frayed end, holding sutures; and (**c**) grade III-C, midsubstance distal (>50%) tear with a severely frayed end, not holding sutures. (courtesy of Ferdinando Iannotti)

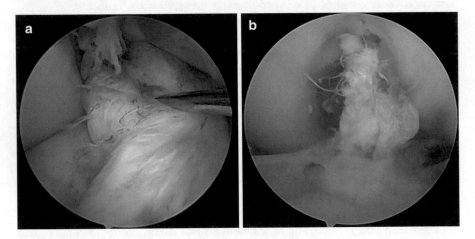

Fig. 14.8 Arthroscopic examples of ACL tears: (**a**) type IA injury (proximal tear with a firm stump); (**b**) type IIIC injury (irreparable ACL tear)

tear type and determine the tissue quality. When it was considered reparable, an accessory anterolateral portal was created, and a 6-mm PassPort cannula (Arthrex Inc., Naples, FL) was inserted. The ACL remnant on the tibial side was prepared by suture passage into the ligament with a knee Scorpion suture passer using no. 2 FiberWire® and TigerWire® stitches (Arthrex Inc.) that were looped through the ligament using a lasso-loop knot-tying configuration. Then, a femoral outside-in ACL guide, placed at the origin of the femoral stump for anatomic guidance, was used to create a femoral tunnel (Fig. 14.9). The femoral tunnel was drilled with a

Fig. 14.9 Femoral drilling of the lateral femoral condyle with an outside-in technique

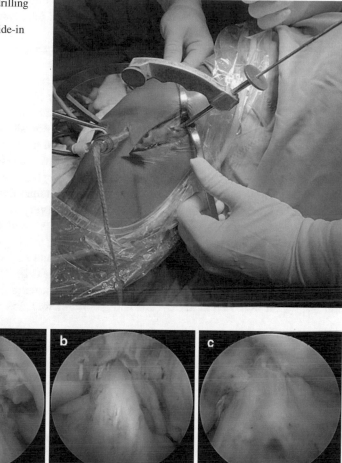

Fig. 14.10 Final arthroscopic views of ACL repairs: (**a, b**) Repair of a type I ACL tear in the right knee; (**c**) Repair of a type II ACL tear in the left knee

3.5-mm drill using an outside-in technique. A FiberStick™ no. 2 (Arthrex Inc.) was then passed through the guide trocar and retrieved with a grasper from the antero-medial portal. The FiberStick™ was then used to shuttle the repair stitches up through the femoral tunnel to reapproximate the tibial ACL remnant to the femoral ACL stump. After cycling the knee, the repair stitches were tensioned with the knee in full extension and then fixed to the lateral femoral condyle with a bioabsorbable 4.75 mm Swivelock (Arthrex Inc.). Finally, the repaired ACL was probed and evaluated at different degrees of flexion to confirm the integrity of the repair (Fig. 14.10). In all cases the lateral compartment was inspected and anterolateral ligament tears eventually repaired, for a more comprehensive treatment of the anterolateral insta-bility in its whole. Recently, other fixation devices using one or two femoral tunnels have been proposed to better restore the functional anatomy of the ACL and to have better repair tension (ACL Repair TightRope®, Arthrex Inc., Naples, FL).

14.1 Postoperative Rehabilitation

A short-ROM knee brace was applied postoperatively for the first 4 weeks. The brace was locked in extension for the first week and then unlocked for the remaining 3 weeks. Weight bearing with braces and crutches was allowed as tolerated on postoperative day 1. The focus of the first week was on pain and swelling control with ice and anti-inflammatory drugs. Range of motion exercises were started 1 week after surgery with the goal of maintaining full extension and progressively recovering flexion. Full ROM was usually obtained by a maximum of 4 weeks after surgery. The brace was removed 4 to 6 weeks after surgery, and patients started a supervised strengthening programme. Sports activities were allowed 6 months postoperatively.

In addition to postoperative rehabilitation, the crucial difference with similar, unsuccessful techniques that we used in the early 1980s (Fig. 14.11) [17] is that at that time, we fully debrided the femoral footprint, removing the whole proximal stumps, which were rich in fibres, cells and growth factors, actually preventing any

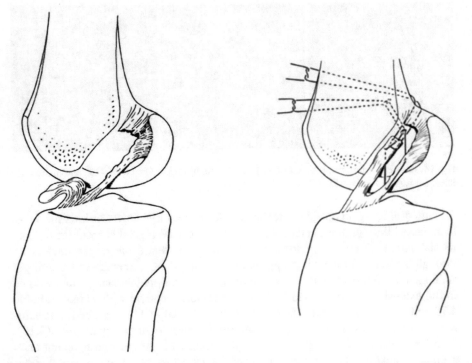

Fig. 14.11 Anterior cruciate ligament repair techniques described by W. Mueller (reprinted with permission from "The Knee," Springer-Verlag ed, Berlin. 1983)

chance of healing. In fact, it was a hopeless attempt to reattach a short remnant to the bone by means of weak, resorbable stitches.

Since the beginning of this new approach for ACL repair, all patients were strictly followed up both clinically and radiologically with sequential MRI performed at 1, 3, 6 and 12 months.

Since 2018, a total of 175 acute (within 2 weeks of injury) ACL surgeries were performed at our institute. Fifty-six patients were excluded because they did not meet the inclusion criteria. Of the remaining 119 patients, a total of 80 acute ACL repairs and 39 acute ACL reconstructions were performed.

In fact, according to the criteria used in this study and the proposed classification for repairability of the ACL, autologous graft harvesting and ACL reconstruction could be safely avoided in more than 60% of the acutely treated cases.

The preliminary results of the sequential MRI study were presented in our first published study [18]. The ACL appearance was classified based on morphology and signal intensity. Morphology was graded as normal (grade 1) or abnormal (grade 2). Signal intensity was compared with the posterior cruciate ligament signal intensity: grade 1 (isointense), grade 2 (intermediate) and grade 3 (hyperintense).

In a total of ten patients who completed the MRI study, there were no early clinical or mechanical failures (the overall IKDC score was graded as A in eight patients and B in two patients). The sequential MRI showed a normal morphology of the repaired ligament at one month in all patients, which persisted at three and six months. Regarding signal intensity, four of the ten patients showed an isointense signal at one month, five showed an intermediate signal and one showed a hyperintense signal. At both 3 and 6 months, the signal intensity was graded as isointense in nine patients and intermediate in one patient (Figs. 14.12 and 14.13).

The main finding of this very preliminary imaging-based study is that the MRI appearance of an acutely repaired ACL seems normal or close to normal in most cases by three months after surgery. These results seem to provide evidence that an

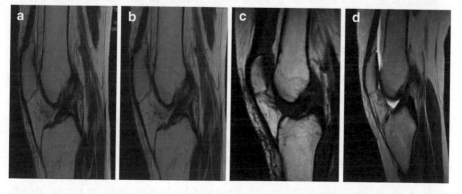

Fig. 14.12 Pre- and postoperative images of an ACL repair. (**a**) Sagittal preoperative MRI T1-TSE; (**b**) Sagittal T1-TSE 1-month post-op. Morphology grade 1 (normal); signal intensity grade 1 (isointense); (**c**): Sagittal T1-TSE 3 months post-op. Morphology grade 1 (normal); signal intensity grade 1 (isointense). (**d**) Sagittal T1-TSE 6 months post-op. Morphology grade 1 (normal); signal intensity grade 1 (isointense)

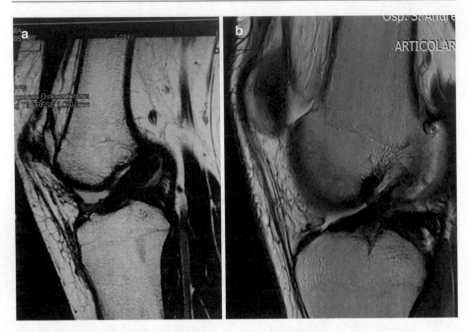

Fig. 14.13 (**a**) Three-month postoperative image of an ACL repair. Sagittal T1-TSE 3 months: morphology grade 1 (normal); signal intensity grade 1 (isointense); (**b**) 1-year postoperative image of an ACL repair. Oblique T2-TSE: morphology grade 1 (normal); signal intensity grade 1 (isointense)

acutely torn ACL, whose stumps can be reapproximated early in tension, has the potential to heal, as revealed by MRI, whose ability to predict the size and mechanical properties of the healing ACL has been proven in a large animal model by the group of researchers led by M. Murray [19].

More recently, we reviewed a much larger number of patients from the above-mentioned prospective study. A more comprehensive clinical evaluation at an acceptable minimum follow-up of 24 months was possible, along with suitable comparison of the reconstruction.

Of a total of 57 patients operated on in the study period, 31 patients had tears that were considered reparable and were repaired, while 26 patients with unrepairable tears underwent standard reconstruction.

Clinically, the mean TLKSS score was 97.56 ($\pm$4.63) in the repaired group and 91.7 ($\pm$10.08) in the reconstructed group; the mean KOOS score was 97.85 ($\pm$2.61) in the repaired group and 93.5 ($\pm$7.05) in the reconstructed group; the mean subjective IKDC score was 96.01 ($\pm$5.12) in the repaired group and 86.93 ($\pm$4.9) in the reconstructed group, with no significant difference between the two surgical procedures. Radiologically, the same group of patients underwent MRI at 1 year postoperatively. Two MRI criteria were evaluated: the signal-to-noise quotient (SNQ) and graft maturity (water content of the graft) based on the Howell scale. The SNQ was calculated with the following formula: SNQ = graft signal – posterior cruciate

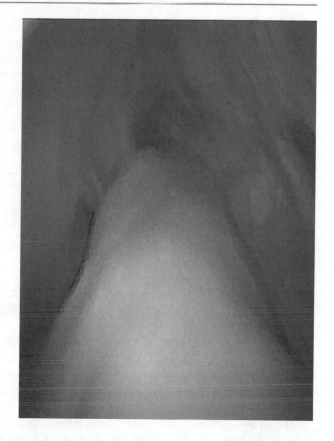

Fig. 14.14 Eight months after ACL repair: second look with needle arthroscopy

ligament signal/background signal. The mean SNQ was 1.96 (±1.04) in the repaired group and 2.52 (±1.7) in the reconstructed group. According to the Howell scale, 22 out of the 31 patients in the repaired group had grade I, 6 patients had grade II and 3 patients had grade III grafts. In the reconstructed group, 19 out of the 26 patients had grade I grafts, 6 had grade II grafts and 1 had grade III graft. As there was no significant difference between the two groups, ACL repair was noninferior to reconstruction either clinically or radiologically. For any surgeon who experiences harvesting-related complications that can occur regardless of the graft used for ACL reconstruction, the advantages of the repair can easily be catch.

In another interesting study that is still in progress, we examined the molecular expression of the repaired ACL compared to the hamstring-reconstructed ACLs. This study was performed in collaboration with the Department of Clinical and Molecular Medicine at our University. Fifteen biopsies were performed during needle or standard arthroscopic second looks between 6 and 12 months after ACL repair (Figs. 14.14 and 14.15). The molecular expression of type 1 collagen, type 3 collagen, alpha smooth muscle actin (alpha-SMA) and the Collagen 1/Collagen 3 ratio were analysed and compared to normal ACL and hamstring-reconstructed ACL. The results of this molecular analysis showed that the repaired ACL is

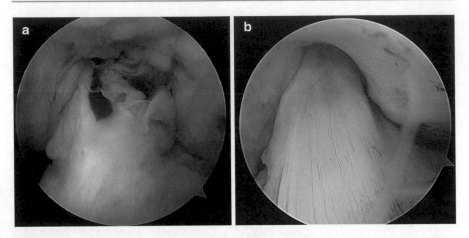

Fig. 14.15 (**a**) arthroscopic second look 10 months after ACL repair; (**b**) arthroscopic second look 1 year after ACL repair

statistically more likely to replicate the native ACL than the reconstructed ACL. Based on these preliminary results, we can reasonably state the following:

- Newly formed tissue after ACL repair is not scar tissue and has biological characteristics close to those of the native ACL.
- The controversial "ligamentization" process of a hamstring-reconstructed ACL is unlikely to be completed up to 12 months postoperatively.

The present technique is based on early surgery performed in the inflammatory phase of the healing process aiming to maximize the potential of healing. The goal of the procedure is to reapproximate the tibial ACL stump to the femoral remnant, which is left "in situ" at the level of the femoral footprint, while they are still at the original length. On both sides, any debridement that could damage the healing potential of the remnants or enlarge the gap should be avoided. Moreover, in any case, repairs should be performed before differentiation towards contractile myofibroblasts occurs, possibly leading to retraction of the stumps and possibly enlarging the gaps.

In our series, there was no augmentation with sutures or scaffolds due to the desire to optimize the favourable healing environment. However, some authors have suggested the use of an internal brace (IB) at the time of ACL repair to protect the biological environment and prevent displacement of the tissue in the healing phase by controlling anterior translation [20]. Other authors, in cases of delayed surgery, have promoted the use of biological scaffolds or stimulation, especially when a shorter retracted stump is found, to optimize the healing environment between the torn ends of the ligament [21, 22]. This technique could be reasonably used when surgery is not performed in the very early stage after injury.

It is thought that proximal tears of the ACL have a better chance of healing than midsubstance injury patterns. In their systematic review, Van der List et al. [15]

showed that indeed, when the historic open ACL repair data were stratified by tear type, patients with proximal tears had better results than those with midsubstance injuries. This is likely due to several factors, including ACL vascularization, as the proximal ACL receives a greater blood supply than the middle and distal third of the ACL. In fact, the site of the tear is one of the two factors considered in our classification system, leading to the final judgement of repairability.

However, even if ACL repair may appear to be an attractive procedure to minimize morbidity and avoid harvesting-related complications, all preliminary outcomes should be considered very cautiously. Moreover, the correct indication in terms of the timing of surgery (acute, subacute and chronic), type of tears (proximal, distal and midsubstance), age, sex, sports activity level, treatment of associated injuries, severity of instability, surgical techniques, augmentation, etc. must be further addressed and possibly elucidated. Whatever the future of ACL repair may be, we must reaffirm that anterolateral instability in ACL-deficient knees is multifactorial and that a more comprehensive surgical approach that is not limited to the ACL is often required, with special attention to the frequently associated injury of secondary restraints and the anterolateral ligament (ALL).

In fact, in all cases when an associated ALL tear is clinically suspected and/or confirmed by MRI, an extra-articular lateral procedure (ALL repair or reconstruction) is performed along with either a repaired or reconstructed ACL procedure.

In any case, it seems easily predictable that other centres and surgeons will soon deal with this challenging topic of ACL surgery and that the issue of ACL repair will become a hot topic of all future meetings and congresses and our team will be there.

References

1. Liljedahl SO, Lindvall N, Wetterfors J. Early diagnosis and treatment of acute ruptures of the anterior cruciate ligament; a clinical and arthrographic study of forty-eight cases. J Bone Joint Surg Am. 1965;47(8):1503–13.
2. Marshall JL, Warren RF, Wickiewicz TL. Primary surgical treatment of anterior cruciate ligament lesions. Am J Sports Med. 1982; https://doi.org/10.1177/036354658201000208.
3. Marshall JL, Warren RF, Wickiewicz TL, Reider B. The anterior cruciate ligament: a technique of repair and reconstruction. Clin Orthop Relat Res. 1979;143:97–106.
4. O'Donoghue DH. An analysis of end results of surgical treatment of major injuries to the ligaments of the knee. J Bone Joint Surg Am. 1955;37-A(1):1–13. passim
5. Murray MM, Martin SD, Martin TL, Spector M. Histological changes in the human anterior cruciate ligament after rupture. J Bone Joint Surg Ser A. 2000; https://doi.org/10.2106/00004623-200010000-00004.
6. Perrone GS, Proffen BL, Kiapour AM, Sieker JT, Fleming BC, Murray MM. Bench-to-bedside: Bridge-enhanced anterior cruciate ligament repair. J Orthop Res. 2017;35(12):2606–12. https://doi.org/10.1002/jor.23632.
7. Trocan I, Ceausu RA, Jitariu AA, Haragus H, Damian G, Raica M. Healing potential of the anterior cruciate ligament remnant stump. In Vivo. 2016;30(3):225–30.
8. Scapinelli R. Vascular anatomy of the human cruciate ligaments and surrounding structures. Clin Anat. 1997;10(3):151–62. https://doi.org/10.1002/(SICI)1098-2353(1997)10:3<151::AID-CA1>3.0.CO;2-X.

9. Spindler KP, Clark SW, Nanney LB, Davidson JM. Expression of collagen and matrix metal-loproteinases in ruptured human anterior cruciate ligament: an in situ hybridization study. J Orthop Res. 1996;14(6):857–61. https://doi.org/10.1002/jor.1100140603.

10. Costa-Paz M, Ayerza MA, Tanoira I, Astoul J, Muscolo DL. Spontaneous healing in complete ACL ruptures: a clinical and MRI study. Clin Orthop Relat Res. 2012;470(4):979–85. https://doi.org/10.1007/s11999-011-1933-8.

11. Fujimoto E, Sumen Y, Ochi M, Ikuta Y. Spontaneous healing of acute anterior cruciate liga-ment (ACL) injuries - conservative treatment using an extension block soft brace without anterior stabilization. Arch Orthop Trauma Surg. 2002;122(4):212–6. https://doi.org/10.1007/s00402-001-0387-y.

12. Kurosaka M, Yoshiya S, Mizuno T, Mizuno K. Spontaneous healing of a tear of the ante-rior cruciate ligament: A report of two cases. J Bone Joint Surg Ser A. 1998; https://doi.org/10.2106/00004623-199808000-00015.

13. DiFelice GS, Villegas C, Taylor S. Anterior cruciate ligament preservation: early results of a novel arthroscopic technique for suture anchor primary anterior cruciate ligament repair. Arthrosc J Arthrosc Relat Surg. 2015; https://doi.org/10.1016/j.arthro.2015.08.010.

14. van der List JP, DiFelice GS. Range of motion and complications following primary repair versus reconstruction of the anterior cruciate ligament. Knee. 2017; https://doi.org/10.1016/j.knee.2017.04.007.

15. van der List JP, DiFelice GS. Role of tear location on outcomes of open primary repair of the anterior cruciate ligament: A systematic review of historical studies. Knee. 2017; https://doi.org/10.1016/j.knee.2017.05.009.

16. Sherman MF, Lieber L, Bonamo JR, Podesta L, Reiter I. The long-term followup of primary anterior cruciate ligament repair. Defining a rationale for augmentation. Am J Sports Med. 1991;19:243–55.

17. Feagin JA Jr, Curl WW. Isolated tear of the anterior cruciate ligament: 5-year follow-up study. Am J Sports Med. 1976;4(3):95–100. https://doi.org/10.1177/036354657600400301.

18. Ferretti A, Monaco E, Annibaldi A, et al. The healing potential of an acutely repaired ACL: a sequential MRI study. J Orthop Traumatol. 2020;21(1):14. https://doi.org/10.1186/s10195-020-00553-9.

19. Biercevicz AM, Murray MM, Walsh EG, Miranda DL, Machan JT, Fleming BC. T2* MR relaxometry and ligament volume are associated with the structural properties of the healing ACL. J Orthop Res. 2014; https://doi.org/10.1002/jor.22563.

20. Massey P, Parker D, McClary K, Robinson J, Barton RS, Solitro GF. Biomechanical compari-son of anterior cruciate ligament repair with internal brace augmentation versus anterior cru-ciate ligament repair without augmentation. Clin Biomech (Bristol, Avon). 2020;77:105065. https://doi.org/10.1016/j.clinbiomech.2020.105065.

21. Gobbi A, Whyte GP. Long-term outcomes of primary repair of the anterior cruciate ligament combined with biologic healing augmentation to treat incomplete tears. Am J Sports Med. 2018;46(14):3368–77. https://doi.org/10.1177/0363546518805740.

22. Murray MM, Fleming BC, Badger GJ, et al. Bridge-enhanced anterior cruciate ligament repair is not inferior to autograft anterior cruciate ligament reconstruction at 2 years: results of a prospective randomized clinical trial. Am J Sports Med. 2020;48(6):1305–15. https://doi.org/10.1177/0363546520913532.

Printed in the United States
by Baker & Taylor Publisher Services